Hit Below the Belt

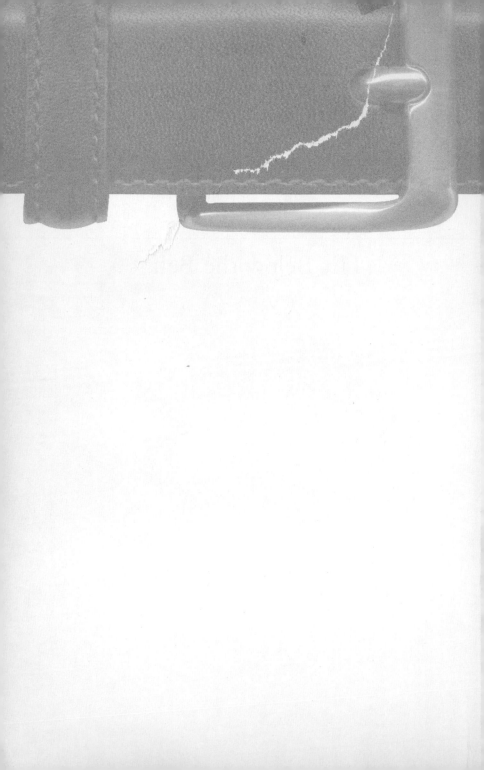

Hit Below the Belt

Facing Up to Prostate Cancer

By F. Ralph Berberich, M.D.

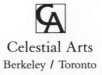

Celestial Arts

Berkeley / Toronto

A Kirsty Melville Book

Celestial Arts
An imprint of Ten Speed Press
P.O. Box 7123
Berkeley, California 94707
www.tenspeed.com

Distributed in Australia by Simon and Schuster Australia, in Canada by Ten Speed Press Canada, in New Zealand by Southern Publishers Group, in South Africa by Real Books, in Southeast Asia by Berkeley Books, and in the United Kingdom and Europe by Airlift Book Company.

Cover and text design by Jeff Puda

Library of Congress Cataloging-in-Publication Data
Berberich, F. Ralph, 1942-
    Hit below the belt: facing up to prostate cancer / by F. Ralph Berberich.
        p. cm.
    ISBN 1-58761-077-9 (pbk.)
    1. Berberich, F. Ralph, 1942---Health. 2. Prostate--Cancer--Patients--California--Biography. 3. Pediatricians--California--Biography. I. Title.

RC280.P7 B47   2001
362.1'9699463--dc21   2001017164

First printing, 2001
Printed in Canada

1 2 3 4 5 6 7 8 9 10 — 05 04 03 02 01

This book is dedicated to my mother, Renee Berberich, and to my father, Leo Berberich, of blessed memory. Together, they fled Hitler's Europe, began a hard, new life in the United States, and gave me life and love. Their example of courage has been a font of strength during rough times.

Acknowledgments

I t will become apparent to the reader that I have taken some pains to respect the privacy of those who have played a role in this story. I did not reveal names in the text and will also not enumerate them here. Nevertheless, I wish to acknowledge those who supported me through my illness. They are all fine people: physicians, family, friends, therapists, members of my synagogue community, rabbis, and colleagues. I thank each and every one of them for their help.

My family deserves special mention. They bore the brunt of my fears and uncertainty, my moods, my intemperance, the times of depression and pessimism. My loving companion, Miriam Petruck, has been steadfast and strong, constantly by my side, and remains ever encouraging. Her quiet integrity and generosity of heart have sustained me throughout. My mother, Renee Berberich, aged and infirm, was a source of profound support and reassurance. My daughter, Jennie, offered me the gift of her youth and optimism, her love and devotion, and the willingness to travel great distances to be with me when I needed her. My family has helped me battle my cancer demons.

Turning to the book itself, I wish to thank my publisher, Kirsty Melville, for offering encouragement and opportunity. My editor, Meghan Keeffe knew just how to balance praise and critique as she guided me through the nuts and bolts of the editing process. She helped revise the manuscript with good cheer and forbearance, displaying a gentle stubbornness that rivaled, even exceeded, my own. Shirley Coe, my copyeditor, had the thankless task of disassembling the first draft, forcing me to render the text more readable, despite my balking at the obvious. My experience at Ten Speed Press demonstrates that authorship can survive moments of literary turbulence and still prove entirely gratifying.

Contents

Chapter One

Introduction

I became a cancer case on July 31, 1998. That was the day I walked into the MRI room, having been assigned a medical record number. I emerged seemingly unchanged, not knowing that cancer would be discovered, that I would be the bearer of a diagnosis, precipitously cast into a pool of like-fated individuals destined to share common paths. Before this time, I had simply been a person who happened to be a doctor, specifically a pediatrician with some prior experience taking care of children with cancer. The transformation to cancer patient was effortless, a passive experience, something that happened to me without my participation and without my being forewarned. I had been given very little emotional lead time. Giving the change little thought, I left one world of experiences and entered another.

This is the story of my unfolding journey, one that overlaps and resonates with stories of roads traveled by others like me. What differs, perhaps, is my perspective as doctor, pediatrician, and former cancer specialist. It is my hope that this book will take the reader away from the customary recitation of facts or messages of unbridled inspiration. What follows is neither a pamphlet to inform the layman, although it contains information, nor a pep talk, although it offers encouragement. Rather it is my own story, told as it unfolded, disclosing what happened to me in some graphic detail, all that I experienced as an individual, my perspective as doctor-become-patient, and some reflections on what I have learned so far from this encounter with life-threatening illness.

I have come to feel that there is great loneliness among men who carry the diagnosis of prostate cancer. The illness arises and is tackled in a male world, one in which feelings are not readily revealed and burdens are often shouldered in isolation. Boys tend not to talk about their feelings. Men are more likely to lock up what they view as personal, and, if they share such matters at all with other men, the exchanges tend to be incomplete or truncated. Sex, family, money, job insecurity, child rearing, conflict, often receive tangential treatment or become jocular, fleeting exchanges. More often, they are suppressed entirely. In a close relationship, they may surface, but most emotions are quickly buried and left to fester within. Perhaps it takes a doctor-turned-patient to share the emotional experience of having prostate cancer, to reveal everyone's sense of vulnerability and fear through his story. It is my hope that this journey will open the hearts and free the tongues of other men with prostate cancer, so the anxiety and pain they carry no longer need be an exclusive burden. I also hope that an open discussion of today's available treatment options, along with one person's convoluted route to his therapy decision, will be of use to others. Above all, we men share a common plight and can profit from each other's experiences.

I begin my tale with some autobiographical details so that the reader can better understand how my experiences colored my thoughts and decisions. I am now fifty-seven years old. I have wanted to be a doctor for as long as I can remember. I can still vividly recall a fantasy I had as a very young child, one that may have kindled my first interest in medicine. I was going to grow up and discover a pill that would allow people to live forever. I would, of course, be among its first recipients. In third grade, I wrote my first medical paper, a two pager that was actually printed in the school yearbook as the literary contribution from my class. I was also featured in a school photograph as Captain Hook, my costume's secret caught in a tangential shot that happened to reveal an open sleeve sheltering a clumsily hidden hand grasping a menacing coat hanger. I think I was more excited by my theatrical experience than I was by my literary achievement. However, it was the essay on the brain that launched my career. "The brain," I wrote, "has two parts, the front part and the back part." On the strength of this illuminating discovery, I progressed onward to medical school.

The father of my best friend was a second influence on my choice of a medical career. A famous plastic surgeon, he traveled all over the world, a towering figure among physicians, the founder of a free clinic in Vietnam devoted to repairing birth defects during the era of exported military destruction. I often heard about celebrities that came his way for some anatomic repair. Surely, I could aspire to no less, and I therefore determined that I should be a surgeon, perhaps even a plastic surgeon. No one could ever accuse me of making rational, rather than emotional, decisions.

The allure of surgery carried all the way through medical school. It was an undercurrent when I had the good fortune to spend a summer working at Harvard Medical School with my cousin's husband, a research anatomist interested in bone marrow cells. Well it wasn't surgery, but I gratefully grabbed the opportunity, and my experience sparked an interest in hematology that was to influence subsequent career choices. During my third year in medical school, the first clinical year, where books gave way to patient contact, I encountered a fine senior surgeon, a pediatric surgeon. This physician had an enormous fund of knowledge, as well as a presence and demeanor that affirmed that pediatric surgery was indeed the most noble and regal of medical fields. In my fourth year, I returned to Boston and did a five-month externship with another well-known surgeon, a cancer surgeon who specialized in removing tumors of the breast, thyroid, adrenal gland, tongue, and mouth, along with anything else that came his way. Once again, this physician and his colleagues at Massachusetts General Hospital dazzled me; their expertise and manner were so distinguished and refined. They were nearly the last of their kind whom I would encounter in the field of surgery.

I had it all planned out: a residency in surgery, then specialization in pediatric surgery. My experience in hematology was an interesting footnote, but I was impatient to be a doer, a fixer, a man of action. What I found as I began my California internship was that I needed to be an early riser, about 5 A.M., a team player with peers I did not respect, a jock, a beer drinker, and a raconteur of off-color and morbid jokes. I was soon disappointed and my discomfort grew with time. My patrician and refined East Coast surgeons were replaced by a group of arrogant cowboys, rough and ready, shamelessly flirting with nurses and chewing the fat, tallying cases like notches in a six-shooter. As my discontent grew, I got into trouble. Things were different in those days. On one occasion, I was strongly advised to manually assist in obtaining the consent signature of an incompetent, elderly gentleman who had been shipped in from a nursing home for an elective hernia operation. The assistance boiled down to taking his hand and signing his name with an X. I refused, a villain then, probably a hero if the same scene were being played today. On another occasion, I was criticized and temporarily suspended because I spent too much time playing with a fifteen-month-old burn patient who needed daily dressing changes, a painful procedure I had to inflict on her. I had become a rebel in surgery and was rapidly developing a bad rep. I came to understand that I was not for these surgeons, and surgery was probably not for me. I have retained both a fascination for and suspicion of surgery ever since that time. This prejudice, and the professional battering from which it emerged, were to follow me into the realm of prostate cancer and color my own response to the diagnosis.

The Chief of Pediatrics heard about me and told me that if I decided not to pursue a career in surgery, he would offer me a slot in the pediatric program, provided I behaved myself. I did not need to be asked twice. And so my career in pediatrics was launched. In the course of my training, I came in contact with a fine pediatric hematologist and began to rekindle that interest. Then as now, hematology, the treatment of blood disorders, and oncology, the treatment of malignancies, formed a single subspecialty. The bridge was leukemia, the most common pediatric malignancy, a cancer of blood cells. Recalling my summer doing anatomic hematology research, I became more drawn to this specialty.

On completing my pediatric residency, I continued with three years of hematology training and research. My first job as a pediatric hematologist came courtesy of Uncle Sam, a career choice I was forced to make once my military deferment expired. At age thirty, I found myself married, living in Seattle, Washington, a major in the United States army, and the Chief of Pediatric Hematology for military dependents in the entire Pacific Northwest. Needless to say, I got my feet wet and learned a bunch. After two years in the army, I began a seven-year stint in pediatric hematology/oncology in California. During this time, along with my colleagues, I had more oncology than hematology experience. Day in and day out, I labored to save children from an early death, watched them respond to treatment, saw some through relapse and dying, saw others grow to maturity, some intact, others missing limbs or faculties. I worked with some oncologists who were inappropriately optimistic and therapeutically aggressive, so I saw the pitfalls of never giving up. I also witnessed the harshness of honesty and reality, even when revealed by compassionate doctors. In the end, I experienced a spectrum of the expected, both favorable and unfavorable, as well as the unexpected cases. Surprises seem to punctuate cancer treatment with teasing and unpredictable regularity. The fickle nature of cancer is never forgotten, even when the particulars of treatment recede into distant memory.

Concurrently, I took on responsibility for the hemophilia program. There was challenging, but good, treatment for this group of bleeding disorders, so curiously, my work in hemophilia became the emotional antidote for disappointments in oncology. These patients suffered a chronic illness, but by and large survived their troubles. It is both sad and ironic that a few years after I left the program, hemophiliacs began to develop AIDS as a result of having received infected blood products. I experienced this tragedy only by learning about my infected former patients secondhand. For me, the treatment of hemophilia remains a completely positive and uplifting experience. I saw nothing other than mastery and an overcoming of obstacles. Many of my patients defied their problem, even took chances, and moved toward normal lives, though they would always run the risk of severe bleeding and bruising.

I left oncology with a personal message, often uttered in semi-jest by the most respected and loved of my mentors: "with cancer, ya never know." I liked this better than the mantra of one of my peers: "Once the crab has you, it never lets you go." Of course at the time, both aroused the smile and chuckle that go with releasing tension and dealing with the depression that accompanies treating chronically sick children. Little did I know how those sentiments would return to haunt me twenty-five years later.

My career took yet another turn when medical politics gave me a choice to remain in the oncology field and begin the academic job moves, or accept an offer from a friend to join her in establishing a new general pediatric practice. I chose the latter, having made a home with my then wife and our two-year-old daughter, settled my widowed mother nearby, and developed a feeling of attachment to my community. So began a twenty-year career as a general pediatrician. It felt as if an emotional weight had been lifted. My new charges were healthy children, not without problems, but offering me a less distorted picture of the medical care of children, one that came to include all those strengths and weaknesses of human character embodied in the family. I became a doctor and advisor to families. I saw joys as well as sorrows. I learned to appreciate that you didn't have to have cancer to need help and significant medical intervention. It was possible to provide meaningful assistance without battling cancer. All problems are problems, and each situation has the capacity to generate a range of worries, some trivial, some profound.

During these years, instead of seeing several patients with leukemia every day, I saw and diagnosed only one case. Fortunately, despite having to endure a relapse and bone marrow transplant, he made it to young adulthood disease free, blessed with a long-term remission. Another child with a life-threatening malignancy also has made it on my watch. A third child, who had a brain tumor, remains in long-term remission and is probably cured, although he has significant impairment from his treatment. I consequently developed two perspectives of cancer: the first seen through the eyes of a doctor in the trenches: the second seen as just another hurdle, one among others, and certainly not one that had to call forth despair.

I returned briefly to the cancer world when I helped care for a friend of mine who had cancer of the esophagus requiring some treatment at home, which I was fortunately able to provide. His bedroom had become a medical mini-treatment node, a little island of cancer hospice care in a neighborhood of normalcy. When I emerged from his house, his plight receded as an aberration. I eagerly, happily, and readily returned to the intense, upbeat lives of the healthy children in my practice. I was no longer an oncologist, just a pediatrician with past oncology experience, one who retained some instincts about cancer. The details were no longer in my grasp, and I saw cancer without the intensity it held for me during that early portion of my career.

However, I felt this altered perspective again when my closest colleague developed cancer of the breast. Suddenly I was once more cast back into oncologist mode, now to help a friend obtain the information she would need to make decisions for herself. I quickly discovered she didn't really need much in that direction, so my pediatric and personal side took over, allowing me simply to assist, encourage, share optimism, and be forward looking. I became just another supportive person in her life. Yet I felt as though I was seeing her through the biopsy, surgery, radiation, and chemotherapy in a way that differed from others. I had a better sense of the whole matter and knew the ropes. It is quite humbling, in retrospect, to realize that this knowledge was actually superficial because it lacked immediacy. I was still playing the role of a doctor in a drama, a person who could mouth the words without having had the personal experience. I thought I knew what I was talking about, but not really, because I knew it as a witness, as an observer, as an unaffected participant. I was not responding from within myself, and my response was devoid of the close-to-the-bone emotions that accompany having that particular disease.

My own diagnosis a year later came as a shock to me. I typecast myself as the doctor in all doctor–patient interactions. This was my persona, and it extended well beyond the medical realm. Being The Doctor in all facets of life has an enormous impact when you are suddenly forced into the role of patient. It can render a doctor-turned-patient among the most difficult of patients. How can you let someone take care of you when you are accustomed to taking care of everyone else? To whom can you relinquish that control? I had so far avoided being on the receiving end. I was not cut out to be a patient, so let's just not do that. Let me simply remain a healthy doctor. My father died of a ruptured aortic aneurysm, a blowout of a major artery, related to heart disease, high blood pressure, smoking, and professional tension in the business world. I thought, actually assumed, that I would eventually suffer a heart attack, hopefully during sleep, and preferably in my eighties or nineties. The possibility that I might have a malignancy or could die from cancer just did not occur to me. The very idea of having cancer seemed unreal.

Yet there it was. I had prostate cancer. With all those men who were neither physicians nor cancer specialists, I now shared the enormity of the physical and emotional concerns that are linked to having a malignancy. In this regard, I was just another patient, another fragile, scared human being, no more, no less. But my fears, my compulsions, my perspective, and my indecisiveness all carried the added weight of my personal history, my past experience in medicine. I would have to learn how to be a patient.

In the course of my illness and treatment, I sought information and comfort from people who shared my problem, from physicians who were experts in prostate cancer, and from journal articles and books. I soon discovered that books and articles generally glossed over the earthy details. The literature on prostate cancer resembles an old-fashioned way of transmitting news about the birds and the bees to children. Before sex ed classes became the rage, teenagers made choices based on information of dubious quality and accuracy supplied by peers or those "What is happening to me?" books. When I read books about prostate cancer, I got the facts, which were presented in dry, clinical fashion and utterly lacking in human understanding. When I read articles in magazines, I got the survivor plus triumph-over-cancer messages. Both were informative but lacked immediacy.

The full impact of treatment goes well beyond facts. It is one thing to read about loss of hair. It's another to see your pubic hair thin to a point you haven't known since before you began adolescence, to see it almost gone . . . to look at yourself while in a public shower surrounded by other men and notice how you have been transformed by your treatment. It's one thing to read that you may lose sexual interest, and it is another to walk down the street, see a gorgeous woman, and have your mind register familiar sexual attraction but only in theory (while another more powerful imposed hormone force repulses any sexual response). You are left feeling that your mind and desires are no longer connected to your body. How can books dealing with the facts of prostate cancer truly relate such sensations? It is like viewing a beautiful painting, sitting by the beach, petting a puppy—all pleasurable and evoking pleasant feelings, but lacking sexual drive and physical attraction. It is one thing to read that hormones may cause depression. It's quite another to note that your every response, even when you are joking or laughing, winds up negative, morbidly pessimistic, doubting, full of self-pity. It is important to learn that despite your conscious effort to be cheerful, this despondency may be present without your awareness. More to the point, it infects those who live with you with unhappiness, a gift you never intended.

Shortly after my diagnosis, I bought a small spiral notebook, my unofficial prostate cancer record, and I have carried it around ever since. This notebook has spent its time either in my briefcase or in my pocket, depending on the stage of consultations or treatment. Whenever any information came my way, I wrote it down in the appropriate section, and I have kept it to this day. There are sections containing pertinent names, addresses, and phone numbers. Another section lists serial PSA results, beginning with the highest pre-biopsy value of 6.1 and ending with the current 0.05. Another section lists the dates of diagnostic tests, while yet a fourth records the dates and types of treatment.

I kept this notebook for a number of reasons. As a doctor, I have often experienced the embarrassing annoyance of having to wing it with the patient in front of me, that is to try to recall something I cannot find in the chart, or something carried out at another medical institution and not contained in the chart at all. Every once in a while, a compulsive parent then bails me out by supplying the missing information, known to her because she kept her own records. Good idea. Further, keeping such a record provided me with some perspective as well as encouragement. Finally, I must confess that it allowed me the illusion of playing doctor in my own case. I was writing in the chart.

Looking over my notebook now, I get an overview of the years of my illness. I see once again that at least a year and a half elapsed from the initial PSA elevation in December, 1997 to the date of the biopsy. I remember that more than a month went by between the positive MRI and the biopsy. I have recorded the period of hormone treatment from October, 1998 through May of 1999. While it seemed like an eternity at the time, looking back at the actual dates helps put this experience in perspective. And of course the date of prostate seeding, May 27, 1999, stands out. The subsequent trail of PSA results begins to resemble a series of illuminations lighting a dark path, each one providing a little more confidence and suggesting that the walk ahead may yet prove both lengthy and fulfilling.

This book, then, is written to imbue the facts of the story with its emotional content and with personal perspective. It is my intent that others will take from it the wherewithal to get through the diagnosis and treatment of prostate cancer with as much equanimity as possible. The material is highly personal and graphic at times. I realized that I would be disclosing information about my body and my personal life, details most people, especially men, tend to keep to themselves, details I am not that eager to share with others. Although I am not secretive, I generally draw the line a little closer than this book would allow. The anonymous reader, however, poses less of a threat than people I know, people who might be affiliated with my medical practice and my own family. Typically my body under my swim trunks has remained a private affair, and the workings of my inner mind were revealed only as I chose to reveal them. Yet this wouldn't be much of a book without such disclosures, so I have had to proceed. This book began as a series of hastily scribbled notes. Later, as I realized that I had something to say to my fellow travelers, I began to organize what I had written, and I developed a list of topics I wished to cover. The development of the book became part of my journey from diagnosis to treatment. These activities have emerged inseparable, as though there had been two of me, one undergoing the experience, and the other taking notes and reflecting on the experience.

People meet me today and ask whether I have completed treatment. I tell them that I have. They then often ask, "So are you a survivor?" or "Are you cured?" or "Does this mean the cancer is gone?" No questions could be stranger when applied to cancer in general and to prostate cancer in particular. To both doctors and laymen, the word "cure" means the illness is over for good. Cancer is never really over unless you die, have an autopsy, and are shown to be cancer free, in which case it is of no interest to you. The passage of time simply reduces the chance of recurrence, but it never completely eliminates it. We therefore speak of remissions, even long-term remissions, but the word "cure" is hardly ever used without understanding its limitations, except by uninformed laymen. Those who know this are mildly irritated when being a cancer "survivor" or being "cured" of cancer becomes the mark of success. It's the same when we encounter the headline "Cancer: The Cure," because we suspect that no single magic bullet will emerge during our lifetimes, or possibly ever. Cancer embodies a wide number of malignancies, each with its own set of characteristics and sites of potential vulnerability to attack. Perhaps someday a unified approach such as gene therapy will govern the basis for treating these malignancies, but it seems unlikely that there will be uniformity or singularity in the treatment. In any event, a magic bullet is so far away that tantalizing announcements and press releases just serve to upset those currently or recently undergoing treatment. Patients have to deal with probabilities, the unknown, and the present, both when we weigh our options and when we measure results. A technical term that reflects this state of affairs is "disease-free survival," a measure of the interval between the end of treatment and the end of the measurement period, relapse, or death from another cause. What a way to gauge the benefit of a treatment!

Yet this is what we have, and we must be content with whatever the art and science of healing provides to fight the disease. In the end, this is a lonely journey no matter what the outcome. Every traveler forges his own path through a thicket of information, decisions, hopes, and consequences. Each of us winds up alone, confronting his mortality and vulnerability. Nothing, not family and friends, nor knowledge, nor level of education, nor money, nor power on earth totally insulates a man or woman from the anguish caused by the threat contained in the word "cancer." I hope this book will soon be factually out-of-date, that newer and better forms of treatment will supplant what is now available. I also hope that a kernel of truth and affirmation and the human factor will endure past this obsolescence and serve its readers well. To all my fellow travelers, I say the words spoken to me by countless colleagues and consultants: *Good Luck!*

Chapter Two

The Saga Begins

Men often slide into the diagnosis of prostate cancer. If they grow old enough, virtually all eventually have it. Yet overall, less than 10 percent of these men die from prostate cancer because so many older people die of other causes. Another important peculiarity of prostate cancer is that it usually grows very slowly, over a period of years, taking a long time to escape the confines of the prostate gland and cause trouble. Thus a man in his seventies may have prostate cancer, sail through his golden years without knowing of the disease, and die from an unrelated cause. Younger men are far less likely to fare as well. Although it is slow to grow for a time, prostate cancer does invariably grow, and if men contract it early enough and live long enough, it will cause grief. For this reason, early detection has become an attractive alternative.

At or around age fifty, men typically begin having an annual screening test for prostate cancer—the PSA (Prostate Specific

Antigen). The PSA screening test is a relatively new development in the detection of prostate cancer. For a long time, physicians relied on a rectal examination of the prostate, the so-called digital exam. This is a nice way of describing the doctor inserting a finger into the rectum and fairly forcefully running that finger over the surface of the gland where it is in contact with the rectum. The search is for protrusions, bumps, or, in medical lingo, nodules. The examination produces some burning discomfort and a feeling that something needs to be allowed to flow out of the penis. Often, a small amount of seminal fluid is pushed out by the pressure of the exam. At the end, just when you are feeling the relief of having that pressure gone, the doctor hands you a tissue so that you can blot away the sticky. It's no fun.

In fact, the rectal exam seems an embarrassing, unpleasant experience from beginning to end, although the whole thing probably takes less than a minute. There is something very infantalizing about it. You have to wipe yourself in public, as it were, exposing at least two emenations we ordinarily take great pains to hide. The usual position assumed for the rectal exam is one you might have experienced if you were ever spanked as a child. Men may quickly surpress the discomfort and vulnerability this exam produces, saying to ourselves that it's nothing, but I have yet to meet anyone who looks forward to it.

Most of urology is no fun when you are on the receiving end. More importantly, the rectal examination is not a very sensitive detector of prostate cancer. Although the area abutting the rectum is the one from which most prostate cancers arise, by the time a distinct nodule of tumor can be felt, there is already a large amount of tumor present in the gland. It was long hoped that a more sensitive test would be developed. But even after the era of the PSA was launched, men were not able to escape the rectal exam. Too bad.

The PSA test has become to men what the mammogram is to women. We live in dread of a result that points to cancer. Like the mammogram, the PSA can give false positive and false negative results. Men whose PSA is elevated may have a normal or noncancerous prostate, while men whose PSA is in the normal range may nevertheless have cancer. To make matters even more confusing, the PSA also rises with age, the size of the prostate gland, prostate inflammation, and a common noncancerous enlargement condition called BPH (Benign Prostatic Hypertrophy). Not only this, but BPH and cancer can both be present in the gland at the same time! Because the PSA is so difficult to interpret, additional tests have been developed to help point in one direction or another.

The PSA comes with no absolute standards describing what is unequivocally normal and what is unequivocally abnormal. Some urologists have lowered their threshold of suspicion and perform biopsies at lower PSA levels than do others. As I looked at the controversy surrounding this test, I began to wonder how our overall results might look if we skipped the PSA altogether and simply performed biopsies on all men over fifty, or on a random number of men chosen by some other criteria. In fact, if prostate biopsy could be rendered as pain-free and routine as the sigmoidoscopy recommended for colon cancer screening, this might be the way to go. The whole PSA issue is so emotionally charged at present, that some men, and even some doctors, shun the test altogether. A friend of mine, a psychiatrist who already had a different kind of cancer, has chosen not to obtain PSAs. He is simply ignoring the possibility of early detection of prostate cancer, preferring that risk to the seemingly endless anxiety imposed by obtaining annual PSAs. Denial can actually be a useful defense mechanism in coping with cancer when judiciously applied. For example, it may help some patients get through radical prostate-ctomy (complete removal of the prostate gland and associated lymph nodes) by denying or minimizing the impact of being bound to a urinary catheter for several weeks, uncertain of the return of continence. However, I am not sure that avoiding the PSA constitutes healthy denial. Prostate cancer does not like to be ignored.

To date, no test short of prostate biopsy reliably and unequivocally determines the presence of cancer. In fact even prostate biopsy, which is unpleasant but can be performed in the doctor's office, may not always give an unambiguous and final result. Because the fine biopsy needles may miss the tumor, some doctors perform more than the customary six biopsies to try to find cancer if it exists. As many as twelve probes may be used to search for that proverbial needle in a haystack. In short, while prostate cancer screening has clearly made a difference by detecting cancers earlier, it remains very problematic, and new techniques are currently being explored in an effort to provide more reliable detection.

Once you embark on the diagnostic path, the whole emphasis is on finding cancer, as opposed to declaring you well. This means that a normal biopsy may lead to the recommendation for repeat biopsy several months later if your PSA is not quite right. This is a pretty abnormal route to diagnosis. Most of the time, when you go to the doctor for an exam or blood work, it is with the assumption that you can get a clean bill of health if all is normal. Now just imagine that instead, your doctor tells you that your tests are all fine, but you should repeat the whole business again in a year to try to find this common problem early if it exists. Some urologists color their to-biopsy-or-not-to-biopsy decisions in one direction or another by using lower trigger thresholds, such as successive PSAs that are in the normal range but rising, or PSAs in the upper range of normal accompanied by a positive family history, or known risk factors such as being African American.

It is very peculiar to undergo a somewhat painful procedure on the basis of a possibly abnormal laboratory test obtained while you feel perfectly fine, and have the process be dedicated to finding even a small tumor that might be present, only to be faced with some pretty unpleasant and uncertain treatment options. In this country, the use of the PSA has been beneficial in detecting cancers earlier, but the test has also generated a whole segment of middle-aged males who must live with its results. If a positive PSA leads to a cancer diagnosis, these men must now ask themselves what to do about their cancer when it is not yet completely clear who needs treatment and who does not. One can understand why some men faced with such a relatively murky scenario might just prefer to take their chances.

In medicine, a pathology diagnosis usually settles matters. What began as a possibility ends as a fact embedded in tissue that has been examined under the microscope. This is not to say that pathologists never disagree or never err. What is viewed under the microscope is subject to interpretation. However, if prostate cancer is present in the biopsy tissue, a diagnosis will likely be made from the specimen. With prostate cancer, a yes or no result is just the beginning. From the appearance of the cancer cells, the pathologist interprets the aggressiveness of the tumor found in each positive biopsy specimen. This interpretation results in a number called the Gleason score, named after the pathologist who developed the scoring system. The Gleason score is extremely important in establishing a prognosis and also figures heavily in the treatment recommendations. As you might think, because it results from an interpretation, different pathologists may assign different Gleason scores to the same specimen. Moreover, the Gleason score obtained at biopsy may differ from that given if the prostate gland is surgically removed and examined as a whole. These number- and score-based determinants can be pretty unnerving. Without getting into too much detail, the Gleason Score (2–10) is reported as the sum of two Gleason Grades (1–5) assigned by evaluating two separate criteria reflecting the degree of tumor maturation, and incorporating sets of features considered either "major" or "minor." The less differentiated (more immature) the tumor, the less it approximates normal cells and glandular tissues in appearance and anatomic pattern. Relatively undifferentiated cancers are considered more aggressive, and aggressive features result in a higher Gleason score. For example, a score of 4 + 3, or 7, indicates a pretty aggressive tumor. The lower the Gleason score, the less ominous the cancer.

In the typical medical setting, a diagnosis comes as a relief and a signal that something definitive can be done. This is not always so, but people get used to the idea that diagnosis and treatment put medical problems in the past tense. Someone will say that he had pneumonia, took Penicillin, and is now cured, or that he had a hernia, had surgery, and is now OK. Other conditions are chronic, perhaps even life-long, but controllable. People afflicted with such a condition learn to cope and live with their problem to the best of their ability. Some illnesses are accompanied by slow deterioration, and people handle this with varying degrees of success ranging from upbeat to deeply depressed.

Cancer is quirky and except in rare cases, the "cure" word must be used with great caution. A malignancy can appear to have been eradicated, only to return with a vengeance years later. Doctors who care for cancer patients typically speak of long-term remissions, rather than cure, and in terms of the statistical likelihood of the disease returning. They use measures like disease-free survival, survival within age brackets, and comorbidity to attempt to judge whether a person is more likely to suffer relapse from the cancer or die from another cause. This is very sobering, putting your mortality and the relative brevity of your remaining lifespan right up there in front of your face. Just as one is diabetic, whether well controlled or not, so one has cancer, a lifelong condition following diagnosis, one fraught with potential complications which never quite releases you while you are alive. A man cannot put prostate cancer entirely in the past tense. He can speak only of the likelihood of its return during the rest of his life.

With cancer, a man is apt to feel that his body has betrayed him, that it has turned against him. An infection invades the body. Beat back the offender and you can be restored. Arthritis and heart disease are relegated to the ravages of aging, the wearing down of a good machine that needs more attention and indulgence to last as long as possible. But cancer cells are our own, misbehaving and rendered deadly, out of control, destroying and distorting us. Beating back the enemy is also beating back ourself.

I began getting PSAs in my early fifties. As is typical for many physicians, I had not had a complete exam for several years. The first test came back showing a PSA level slightly above normal. The decision was to do another test in a few months after taking precautions against activities that could falsely elevate the result of the test. The second PSA was slightly lower. Six months later, it was slightly higher. And so it went, hovering between a value of 4 and 5 for a year and a half. My rectal exams were all normal, and I felt as well as a busy pediatrician ever feels. Finally, my internist suggested I see a urologist, who was as gentle a friend and colleague as one could hope for. Of course, I knew that referral to a urologist in this setting meant I would receive a recommendation to perform a biopsy. In my own pediatric practice, I refer patients to surgeons for one of two reasons. Either I have already determined that an operation is required, or I am uncertain and desire a surgeon's opinion. I do not refer if I am convinced that surgery is not necessary. This would be a waste of the surgeon's time. It is slightly different for a urologist, who treats many conditions noninvasively, but not in the setting of an elevated PSA.

The word biopsy generated such fear and foreboding that I actually convinced my urologist to delay a few more months. The fear of pain in "that" area ranked high, but I also had this notion, not completely imaginary or hysterical, that putting a needle through a little tumor could spread the cancer. What I did not know was that any tumor cells dislodged during a biopsy do not

seem to settle in other sites, but rather they simply die. This phenomenon, called apoptosis, is intriguing because it says something
about the nature of early prostate cancer, but it bears little on the
unfolding of this part of the story. Perhaps it mostly illustrates
once again that knowledge and past experience cannot always be
transferred to a new situation. If it leads to false conclusions, such
knowledge can actually be a hindrance. Had I known about the
peculiar properties of loose prostate cancer cells circulating in the
body, I might have been more eager to have the biopsy earlier.

So, swayed a little by my reluctance, my urologist ordered a
total and "free" PSA, which is thought to help distinguish between
benign and malignant causes of elevated PSAs. Most PSA circu-
lates in the blood bound to protein, but PSA from cancer cells
breaks loose from the protein, therefore circulating as "free"
(unbound) PSA. My results were not reassuring. They suggested
I might have cancer. Still seeking to avoid biopsy, I started down
the long road of personal research and discovered that the local
university center had embarked on a very sophisticated form of
prostate MRI that could accurately inform a physician about the
likelihood of finding cancer.

Let me pause here to describe the pecking order in the medical establishment. Most general and specialist physicians work in
a private practice or clinic setting. Some are solo practitioners,
while others work in groups, sometimes embodying a single specialty or, in the case of larger clinics, a group representing many
specialties. Some of these large groups have international reputa-
tions for excellence and innovation, while others are simply col-
lections of well-qualified doctors. Other groups of subspecialists
band together to form medical institutes devoted to treatment of

a single condition or group of conditions. Doctors that are hospital based are considered in many circles to be a notch up because specialists at a hospital may have greater experience with a particular illness or group of illnesses. And at the theoretical top of the pyramid are the university hospital specialists who provide so-called tertiary care, the third deepest level of complexity. These doctors characteristically have academic appointments and medical staff privileges. This means that they typically are expected to conduct research, thereby attracting more, and perhaps more difficult, cases in their chosen specialty or subspecialty. You are apt to find your primary care doctor in the private sector, who will then refer you to a urologist, either in private practice or hospital based, who may or may not refer you to a prostate specialist, a more specialized urologist, or a radiation therapist, either hospital or university hospital based. There is a tendency, especially among doctor-patients, to head for the top. It is assumed that university or large clinic/institute physicians know more about your condition and are more experienced and successful in its treatment. That assumption may or may not be justified. The risk in taking this direction is that of less personalized treatment. The more rarified and unique the specialist, the greater the tendency for you to be one among many, a research subject or cipher.

In the summer of 1998, I chose to have the ultra-specialized MRI at the university medical center. It seemed the least invasive of alternatives, and I thought it would show nothing. I was strangely on my own arranging to have this MRI. I located one of the authors of the research paper I had read, chatted with him, heard his glowing reports about the accuracy of the study, and made an appointment. My case actually generated some excitement, because I became a piece of valuable data. Most men have these prostate cancer-specific MRIs after a biopsy, complicating the interpretation. Mine was to be a virgin prostate, free of bleeding or other artifact.

I understood I was not undergoing a standard accepted procedure when I was directed away from radiology and the main clinical MRI section to a separate wing of the hospital. After a series of false turns, I found a research MRI unit solely devoted to this study. I had already been given some dietary instructions, which I had followed, and instructions for an enema, which I had half followed. I now found myself sitting in the waiting area with an older gentleman, who had relapsed after surgery and had undergone a number of these studies to follow the success of his secondary treatment. This was the first of a series of face-to-face encounters I had with people who now constituted prostate brethren, with whom I was cast in a weak bond, and from whom I tended to separate myself, hoping and thinking that my case would be different.

I knew about the isolation and boredom of MRIs, but the experience surpassed my expectations. The technician had me lie on my side while he placed a plastic probe up my rectum to mark its location relative to the prostate. My rectum suddenly felt full as though I had to have a bowel movement for an hour. But amazingly enough, I adjusted to it and quickly reached a state of equilibrium in which I knew the probe was present, but suppressed the feelings its presence created. I then lay on my back, strapped onto the gurney to eliminate motion, a headset and classical music provided for my sanity. The technicians told me the number and length of periods during which I would be entombed in the MRI

chamber and forewarned me about noises—grinding and clunk-
ing that would accompany the working of the magnets. While
these sounds may be disquieting, and the entire study disturbing
to those inclined toward claustrophobia, I remained fairly comfortable throughout knowing nothing would hurt, nothing was
being cut, and no radiation was being transmitted to my body.
The most irritating part for me was that the sound quality of the
music was awful and the sound level was unpredictable. Although
Rachmaninoff's second piano concerto would not have been my
first choice for this experience, I did not find the piece loathsome:
I knew it well and might have been able to follow it from beginning to end, blotting out the rest of what was occurring. Instead,
I heard Rachmaninoff plus clunks plus static as a mélange of noise
forming more of an annoyance than a distraction. Never mind.
It ended, as all these things eventually do, and another technician
slipped the probe out, rendering me a free man once again. The
research investigator with whom I first had spoken emerged,
beaming, and said that mine was a beautiful study. I felt certain
that this meant it looked clear to him, but he quickly added that
no results would be forthcoming until it was completely analyzed
and carefully read by the physician in charge. The façade of camaraderie, the one that suggests, Come on, we're all docs here, just
let me in on what you see, completely evaporated.

I began what remains one of the most tension-arousing states
that characterizes this whole business: waiting for results. Be it a
study, a biopsy, a PSA, or what have you, waiting for results is
nerve racking. A patient knows that whatever is there simply is,
and has been for some time. The study will only disclose the truth,
not create it. Yet the mind plays tricks on you, and you imagine

that positive thoughts or prayers can somehow magically change something bad into something good. I suppose this magical wishing and thinking is part of human nature, yet I blush inwardly each time it happens. I waited and waited. Over a week went by. Eventually I heard from my shocked urologist the same day I received the report in the mail as though I were the referring physician. The MRI definitely suggested tumor, and a lot of it. The only good news was that there was no evidence of spread beyond the anatomic capsule enclosing the prostate gland.

I was devastated and frightened beyond words. From having read the research papers, I knew I now had a 96 percent chance of having cancer of the prostate. The only question now was, how bad? On the game board of this process, in which the end is so undefined, my piece had just moved forward. I was destined to have a biopsy now, like it or not. My urologist tried his best to be positive and reassuring, and he suggested I have the expert at the university medical center perform the deed. I called to schedule the event, only to learn that this physician was abroad and that I would not have the procedure for six weeks. Everyone thought I would go nuts waiting, but I was secretly relieved to have the respite.

Meanwhile, I obtained copies of the MRI and these became my calling card, my exhibit that I lugged around everywhere and showed everyone. A friend of mine is a radiologist who lives in the world of CT scans and MRIs. Once, when he was at my house, I showed him the films. Sure enough, he pointed out to me, holding films up to the incandescent ceiling light, there it was, not even subtle. I carried those films like a portfolio, my innards on display. Now that it is all behind me, the MRI sits in my bedroom closet perched on top of my clothes, a strange place for an X-ray folder. But where else would I store it? And could a doctor bring himself to discard his own MRI? Hardly. So there it remains for all time, like an exhibit in a museum, to be a reminder of something in the distant past, unpleasant, but gone.

I used the interval between the MRI and the biopsy to worry and also to try to learn whether there were special tests that could be performed on the upcoming specimens, all twelve of them. New biochemical and genetic markers were indeed being identified, but not at the medical center conducting my biopsy. Such markers identify specific characteristics of cells. In some cases they can show metabolites that are associated with malignancy. In other examples, the presence or absence of certain markers indicates a different prognosis, or susceptibility to certain kinds of treatment. In the end, since all the local clinicians and prostate experts maintained that getting experimental markers would have no impact on my treatment, none were sought. I also had this idea that some of my tissue ought to be saved, frozen, not pickled in preservative for microscopic viewing, just in case new tests emerged in the future. In particular, some new research was focusing on the presence or absence of p53, a regulator gene that could be prognostically important. But looking for p53, also, was not to be. It is often difficult to coordinate medical studies or tests between major medical institutions. This is especially true when clinical laboratories and individual physicians have their own way of doing things and when a physician is a star in his or her field. After I met the man who subsequently performed my biopsy, I had the sense that there was no purpose in suggesting anything different from his routine unless the rationale was truly compelling. He was the expert, and I was decidedly in his hands. My speculations and theories would likely not be of any great interest to him. His stake was in the accuracy of diagnosis, and then his job was done. I did not think he would suffer fools gladly, so I demurred.

The six weeks of waiting passed. It was time for the biopsy. The treatment areas at the university medical center are small cubicles. One is very conscious of space constraints. Great views of the Golden Gate Bridge, but not much space for anything else. A nurse showed me into a room that housed only a tiny desk, an exam table, an ultrasound machine, and a cart upon which I readily spied vials of preservative and some nasty-looking long needles. My biopsy physician entered and we spoke amiably for a few minutes, after which he asked that I undress and lie down on the table, curled up on my left side. Despite my having taken both analgesics and narcotic medication, I was fully alert, heart racing, tense, and mentally ready to run out the door. I stayed put, of course, as he returned and quickly and efficiently began applying lubricants and anesthetic cream inside my rectum. I had been told that this physician uses an anesthetic local injection before doing the actual biopsies. Not all doctors do, for reasons that escape me, especially after having had the procedure. I was adequately forewarned. The first injection would sting, but I needed to hold still.

I knew pretty much what was coming, of course. My rectum was now personally established as the portal of entry to my prostate from the outside world. It gave the simplest and closest access to the area of concern without doing any cutting. Here is where tubes, probes, needles, were destined to go. Naturally, the more often things were shoved up there, the more sensitive I became to the sensations that accompany that pleasure.

As the needle penetrated my rectum into the prostate, it stung a lot. In fact, it hurt like hell. I was not inclined to hold still, and there was a sharp remonstration combined with a reminder about the delicacy of the anatomy presently exposed to a long needle. I held still. There were two additional injections of anesthetic, each more bearable than the one preceding. In pediatrics, we often buffer the anesthetic with sodium bicarbonate to reduce the sting. I think adult medicine is less concerned with what is thought to be minor, or short-lived pain, as though a grown person ought to enjoy or endure pain more than a child. I see no virtue in any physical pain, especially now, and I heartily endorse any interventions, no matter how small or inconvenient, that safely reduce pain.

Once the anesthetic took effect, my experience became quite bearable. I felt a little snap with each of the twelve biopsies, but they did not hurt. It was only my mind that couldn't wait for the whole thing to be over. When it was over, having taken less than ten minutes, the vials were each labeled, combined, and bagged for pathology. I was told to expect bleeding in my urine for a short period of time and blood in my semen for weeks, depending partly on the frequency of ejaculation. The doctor's delivery was quite brisk and matter of fact. I left offering the expected polite gesture of the Good Patient, thanks and gratitude proffered to the one who did the deed, and I said the expected complimentary words signifying that the whole thing hadn't been too bad an experience. Truth to tell, except for that first injection and my fear and anticipation, the remainder had been quite tolerable.

Pieces of my prostate were now in a brown bag, handed back to me for transport to pathology. I was not in great pain, just a bit sore. I negotiated the elevators and corridors to the designated station and waited in the lines that characterize large institutions. I deposited my specimen after ensuring beyond a doubt that it was correctly identified and headed to the right place. As a physician, I had been the victim of lost patient specimens many times. No way was this going to happen to me as a patient. I had parked down the street a bit, rather than in the hospital garage, just to be macho and contrary. As the anesthetic began to wear off while I was walking downhill, I felt as though someone had kicked me in the butt. The ache was not severe, but it was deep and disquieting. I was happy to sit down in the car. No sooner did I feel relief over the completed biopsy than I began to worry about the findings. How bad would it be? Was I destined for surgery despite my fears?

I had been told to expect results in a few days, but the days passed, one after the other, soon exceeding a week. I was collecting professional cards by now, and the one with the biopsy urologist's name and number sat on my desk at work. Every day, I would get my hopes up for a personal phone call with some good news. The tension mounted, yet I expected to be able to carry on at work, taking care of my little charges with their teddy bears and minor ills as though all was well. I have no recollection of home life at that time, but I'm sure I was no fun to be around. I finally reached the busy urologist, and he blurted out the findings quickly, not without compassion, yet professionally removed, just as I am when I deliver bad news. Not too good, he said. All biopsy sextants (all six sections probed) were positive for cancer, to varying degrees. Because I had an area the pathologists read as 4 + 3, my Gleason Score was a 7. Elsewhere, I had 3 + 4, also a score of 7, but a smidge more favorable. There was a nodule located where he, the only urologist who thought my digital exam abnormal, had felt a bulge. Before the biopsy, he had been talking surgery. Now, he said, maybe radiation would be a better course. That should have been a relief, given my fear of surgery, but of course, the news was frightening because of its implications.

When a tumor is relatively small, it is said to be operable, providing the surgeon can reach and excise it. This means that it is possible to remove the tumor entirely. When applied to prostate cancer and early detection, the implication is that a small, operable tumor *should* be removed surgically. A small area of cancer contained within the gland seems like the perfect scenario for surgical removal, and it is in this setting that the success of an operation is greatest. Indeed, were it not for the associated complications, this would be every prostate cancer patient's dream, namely hope for a small tumor that can be taken out. One would wish to catch the cancer at its earliest stage precisely so that it could be removed along with the gland that spawned it. Once the area of cancer has increased, the chance of surgical eradication diminishes, and the techniques recently developed to spare the nerves that enable sexual function, are rendered moot. For many men, just the hope that the cancer can be removed is sufficient to wish for an operable tumor, despite the surgical risks and complications involved. Others who are more leery of surgery have a mixed response to a prostate expert's endorsement of radiation as opposed to surgery. On one hand, we may be relieved not to have to confront the decision, but we also are frightened by the likelihood of spread of the disease to a point where surgery is deemed not curative.

Not knowing what to say, I simply thanked the urologist and hung up the phone devastated. I don't remember whether I cried or not. I did speak with my personal urologist who tried to be as reassuring as he could. I called my partner at home. I'm sure both of us wept and suffered.

Our sense of tragedy was undoubtedly increased by one of those peculiar convergences that make you wonder about justice in the world. My partner was diagnosed with cancer of the endometrium the same day I was first diagnosed with cancer of the prostate. She had gone through an extensive period of bleeding, symptoms, examinations, biopsies, and protracted hormonal manipulations. Now she faced, and subsequently underwent, a hysterectomy. For two previously healthy people, all of this just seemed like too much. There was no equanimity for either of us. The unexpected blow stressed our unity beyond measure. One wants simply to come together at such times, but the fact of two stressed and scared people living together has its own inescapable implications.

The next hours and days are vague in my memory. I don't remember whether I slept, ate, or answered the phone. Our local hospital now had on staff its own prostate cancer specialist, a radiation oncologist who had trained at the regional medical center and was reputed to be both excellent and kind. I put in a call to him and he called me back quickly, saying he would see me the following day. I am sure that my linking up with this physician helped me through the first days of shock and disbelief. He was extraordinarily kind. But the timing of everything else remains a blur in my mind. At some point, I called my daughter, who was living abroad, and told her the bad news. I also told my eighty-nine-year-old mother, who either absorbed the information incompletely and without its full implications, or had the wisdom not to reveal the level of her understanding.

My consultation with this first of many prostate specialists was an experience in optimism. He felt his digital rectal exam of my prostate was normal and did not get terribly excited about the comments of the urologist who had performed the biopsy. He was very encouraged by the absence of signs of spread on the MRI. He pointed out that my PSA was still low. The entire prostate was not heavily involved. The size of the gland itself seemed relatively small on exam, rendering treatment easier.

At the end of the meeting, he laid out an array of therapy options including: surgery; a mini-surgical procedure to sample lymph nodes followed by radiation; external beam radiation alone, at a variety of doses and by a variety of different techniques, either limited to the prostate or encompassing the whole pelvis; external beam radiation, prostate or whole pelvis, plus radioactive seeds; short-term hormone administration plus radiation; and "watchful waiting." The last possibility was the only one he immediately dismissed as unwise. He felt that cure, in the sense of indeterminate, long-term remission, was still a strong possibility and that I should go for it. When I stated that I did not see surgery as the best choice, he did not object. I left feeling somewhat encouraged, my head spinning from the various choices and possible treatment combinations dumped in my vulnerable lap. I knew that the first step had to be a search for metastases, or cancer spread, to the bones. If the tumor was shown to have spread, most of the options were moot. Knowing the chances for such spread were extremely low, I nevertheless palpably felt fear as I picked up the phone and scheduled the bone scan.

Bone scans are not particularly frightening or uncomfortable. Accustomed to getting off on the third floor of our hospital, where the postpartum beds were located, I had to think twice to press four and get off on the right floor. Nuclear Medicine was set off the main corridor and looked like a fairly harmless collection of cubicles with scanning machines, each surrounded with curtains for a modicum of privacy. I received an intravenous injection of radioactive tracer, one that settles in bones. It was strange realizing that my blood was being nuked, but I knew that the dose was very small, much smaller than what my body was destined to receive during any radiation treatment. In any event, I had little choice. I was subsequently free for two hours, time for the isotope to be absorbed by the bone. I returned after lunch, stretched out on another cot, hooked up a headset, and was delivered, conveyer belt-style, into a scanner, which methodically surveyed my long bones. I was at rest now, ironically confined and prevented from my routinely frenetic daily pace for an hour and a half. Because motion would invalidate the study, one has to lie still, something we imagine to be easy, but actually quite challenging. All the clichés hold true. I wanted to scratch my nose, scratch the itch on my toe, have my aching back massaged. Eventually, as was to become the pattern, this too came to an end. I left the Nuclear Medicine area, once again transformed from subject to the man in waiting, relegated to the tension of uncertainty, hope, and fear.

A couple of days later, I learned that my bone scan was negative. The physician who had read it was a long-time colleague in internal medicine, someone with whom I had casual chats in the halls, another doctor with a hematology background. I'm not sure he ever realized that it was my bone scan he had signed. He was not the one who called with the results. I subsequently told him of my diagnosis, and he seemed surprised because I am about ten years his junior. Less than a year later, he too was diagnosed with cancer.

My work-up was now as complete as I thought reasonable, given my up-front preference to avoid surgery. The statistical chance of lymph node spread was less than 10 percent in my case. Seminal vesicles could not be sampled by mini-surgery. Negative sampling, in any event, could not entirely exclude their involvement. I was done with the first part of the journey. I had adenocarcinoma of the prostate, moderately undifferentiated, Gleason score 7, extensive bilateral involvement of the gland, a low PSA of 6.1, and no evidence of extension beyond the prostate, but a high statistical risk that tumor had already penetrated the gland's capsule. I was still a person, of course, more than just a case, but I was now defined by my staging as far as my treating physicians were concerned. The stage of cancer is a way of describing the known degree of involvement, basically local and confined, as opposed to regionally or distantly invaded. I was also destined to become an anecdote, in the sense that I was not going to be enrolled in any study or therapy trial. The success or failure of whatever treatment I was to choose would be of absolutely no use to anyone else. What remained was to select therapy to best match the level of tumor involvement, a task I now understood was my choice among many equally plausible options.

I knew my approach would be painstaking and protracted. Although professional decision making comes easily to me, I am slow to make decisions for myself. In addition, I had discovered that I required a self-directed compulsive research effort. I needed to complete an exhaustive probe of the subject as a coping mechanism to address my anxiety. This was to be my personal effort to control the uncontrollable. The research would both arouse and allay fear. Both I and my family would be tried and exhausted by the process, and it was to drag out for months.

Chapter Three

Entering the Maze

D espite being frightened and a bit bewildered, a prostate cancer patient must face up to a series of choices, weighty decisions that determine the path he will take. What follows here is a distillation and overview of these options and a smattering of information about each of them. Some themes and facts are repeated later, as my own story unfolds, and this is entirely fitting. The process of arriving at decisions typically is not a simple or straight path. Considerations temporarily laid to rest often reemerge, especially when raised by yet another consultant, perhaps in a slightly different light the second or third time around. Each expert's opinion both builds and meshes with the previous ones, sometimes clarifying matters, sometimes confusing them, sometimes seeming to lead toward consensus, and sometimes seeming contradictory. Denial, vacillation, fear of the unknown, may all distort what is presented, altering what the prostate cancer patient hears. Repetition also helps the person who is learning about this malignancy, because the amount of information can be daunting, even overwhelming, the first time it comes around. I, too, first heard a litany of choices, and then reviewed each in painstaking fashion, adding information along the way and being exposed to the same facts and opinions again and again.

The typical medical model for treatment starts with a complaint, termed a symptom, or with a physical finding detected by either the patient or the doctor. An examination is done, followed, depending on findings, by X rays, lab work, fancier tests, and finally, a diagnosis. Most of the time the doctor prescribes a course of treatment based on the diagnosis. If the diagnosis involves any complexities, a specialist may enter the case, only to repeat the process. As technology has advanced, the involvement of specialists is ever more the rule than the exception, and it sometimes leads to conflicting opinions. A variety of treatment options may yield a single recommendation on the part of each doctor, but it leaves the ultimate choice up to the patient. The patient, of course, may be the least equipped emotionally and intellectually, to render a decision truly in his or her best interest when faced with a diagnosis of cancer. Sometimes the original physician, a family practitioner, or internist, helps guide the patient. Sometimes the decision is based on a gut feeling in reaction to a consultant, a sense of trust or mistrust. These are not necessarily the best means open to a vulnerable person facing a tough life choice.

This emotional quandary is clearly evident with prostate cancer patients. These days, the first step toward diagnosis is likely to be an abnormal PSA obtained as part of a routine checkup. Men who are having their PSAs checked routinely either for diagnosis or after treatment to identify potential relapse may become psychological slaves to this test. They anticipate results with fear and foreboding. Little blips up or down on their numbers take on tremendous significance. This is especially frustrating knowing that the PSA can be abnormal when cancer is absent and normal when cancer is present.

Let us now return to our man who has had his first suspicious, elevated PSA screen. At some point, assuming the PSA remains abnormal, either the patient or doctor will become sufficiently nervous to proceed to the next step. The patient now enters a common pathway we can call the prostate cancer workup. Although new techniques are being developed to try to distinguish cancerous from noncancerous prostate conditions, as of this writing, prostate biopsy remains the ultimate next step, the only definitive diagnostic tool.

Once the biopsy has been completed, and the patient leaves the urologist's office, he has to cope with waiting for the verdict. Some people are able to put the tension behind them, saying that whatever is there has been present for some time. Others find these days excruciatingly painful.

Once a positive diagnosis is established, the person with the cancer, now a patient, begins a journey down a number of professional pathways when the diagnosing doctor, typically a urologist, tells him there are basically three options from which to choose: radical prostatectomy, that is, surgical removal of the prostate; radiation; and watchful waiting. The lay pathway, by contrast, is remarkably multirouted, with friends, relatives, and even strangers, telling you what attitude you should have, how you should feel about cancer and its treatment, and how you should manage your life in general. They may suggest a variety of "alternative" treatment approaches.

Without being skeptical about "alternative medicine," the term is charged and carries with it some assumptions that need to be questioned. By incorporating the word "medicine," alternative medicine is grouped together with the rest of medicine, suggesting they are but limbs of the same tree. Traditional medicine and alternative medicine actually have little in common other than the shared intent to achieve healing. Alternative healing can range widely from herbs to diet to vitamins to acupuncture to homeopathy to chiropractic to massage to visualization to meditation, yet still remain linked to traditional medicine in the mind of a layperson.

Including alternative approaches in the standard medical model is furthered by their incorporation into insurance reimbursement and managed care systems. Some skeptical people would even suggest that alternative therapies are more attractive to insurers, because they are less costly. Yet the basis for knowledge and treatment in these two health care systems is not the same. One is based on slowly accumulated evidence, generally using a painstaking and body-oriented scientific approach. Being more scientific, by the way, does not necessarily mean being more correct. Alternative approaches tend to be experiential, individualized for each case on a less rigorous basis, and more often directed as much toward the mind as toward the body. The standard medical model tends to produce interventions that have side effects. The alternative model is formulated differently. It purports to produce interventions that build and utilize the body's own defense mechanisms to promote health.

Because it sounds, and often is, less invasive, and because the word "alternative" suggests potentially better, cancer patients often find alternative (or complementary) medicine attractive. Think about the word: Alternate routes suggest less traffic; an alternative method suggests a better choice than what is familiar. An alternative approach to treatment implies a secret and less threatening path to healing and restored health. Alternative medical treatments especially appeal when standard approaches don't offer great cure rates. It seems reasonable to seek an alternative on one's own as opposed to being told to have standard treatment, especially treatment frought with the risk of unpleasant complications. Proponents of alternative medicine and holistic healing inspire faith in the body's own natural defense mechanisms and recuperative powers. Small wonder that many cancer patients have as much or more faith in these approaches as they have in "regular" medicine.

If alternative approaches are seen as being unproven, can we rely on logic to formulate medical treatments? Most honest medical practitioners will confess that cold logic also has pitfalls and cannot always predict the specific results of cancer treatment. That which seems as though it ought to work does not necessarily prove successful. Therefore, most medical outcomes, especially those targeted at cancer, need to be judged on the basis of randomized clinical trials. Ideally these are also conducted in double blind fashion: Two rigorously chosen pathways, usually testing an established form of treatment against a more experimental one, are tested by randomly assigning similar patients to one or the other. Furthermore, those conducting the trial do not know which patients have been chosen to receive which treatment.

The effectiveness of a treatment can only really be assessed in this manner. Without such trials, untested logic carries no more weight than faith. In fact treatment based on logic alone relies on a faith of its own, the faith that human reasoning really mirrors the body's reality.

When logic is invoked in my pediatric practice, I often cite the following example to show how it can fail us: logic would predict that nasal decongestants given to a child who has a cold should prevent ear infections. But every time this logical assertion has been tested, no positive effect has been found. Unfortunately, we just are not as smart as we think we are. We often learn that things actually are not as they appear to us, but only if we test our theories with care.

Yet alternative approaches, often supported by attractive reasoning and logic seem attractive. Since they are not shackled by rigorous evidence-based requirements, they tend to come to popular attention quickly and convincingly in accordance with testimonials. "I know someone who did/took X and he's fine now," is a theme that will dance before you like a beckoning siren. Over and over, well-meaning people with absolutely no expertise in prostate cancer will encourage you to seek out an alternative approach—a special drink, a healer, a prayer. None of these approaches is necessarily harmful or bad. Some may eventually be shown to be beneficial. You may partake of an alternative approach that appeals to you and causes no harm. It is important to realize, however, that herbal remedies—often imported from other countries, typically not subject to rigorous controls, and largely unstudied—may not be safe and may cause irreversible damage, much like conventional drugs. Until alternative treatments are supported by evidence according to the standard medical model, they should not be considered an established part of medicine, and they should not be approached casually.

Unfortunately, the traditional medical model also fails those of us facing prostate cancer, at least to a certain degree. It takes many years of evidence-based research, sometimes ten, fifteen, or even twenty years, before a definite conclusion can be drawn. This is because the disease evolves so slowly that a person previously thought cured can relapse many years after treatment. Also, after some forms of treatment, minor fluctuations in the PSA are hard to interpret. To some they represent local failure of treatment. To others, small increases may even indicate a good prognosis. Anway, what is the meaning of PSA-detected local relapse when the goal of treatment is to have you survive long enough to die from something else? What a bizarre way of looking at illness! We just want to be free of prostate cancer. The traditional medical approach rests on thin ice because most of us who have been diagnosed with prostate cancer feel we cannot afford to wait years to find out if a particular form of therapy is eventually going to prove effective and worthwhile.

The medical model is further handicapped by the understandable reluctance of patients to submit to comparative studies testing one treatment form against another. Can you imagine deciding between surgery and radiation by the flip of a coin? Finally, and not insignificantly, doctors invest their careers and grants in particular therapies, and are therefore very biased toward those treatments.

In the treatment of early prostate cancer, there really are no neutral experts. Surgeons lean toward surgery, while radiation therapists lean toward radiation. Those who do seed implantation recommend this treatment and devote lifetimes to improving it. Thus your treatment choice may well depend on the presentation and eloquence of a particular expert, more than on absolute fact.

Knowing that many older men develop prostate cancer, but few die of the disease, makes it tempting to do nothing about your condition. This is the "watchful waiting" option in which serial PSA tests track the cancer's progress, trying to discern whether and when you might get into trouble if nothing definitive is done. It is very tempting to go this route when you feel fine and there is no guarantee of a better outcome with invasive treatment. On the other hand, we do know that early detection and treatment of prostate cancer has reduced the death rate significantly. So what to do becomes a numbers game with the decision as much matched to your needs and desires as to some absolute medical dictum. Furthermore, in the end, no matter what therapy option is chosen, we must return to watchful waiting as the only measure of the treatment's success.

Cancer treatment differs from any other. To begin with, it hardly ever makes you feel better. In fact, people often feel fairly well when cancer is diagnosed. It becomes an act of will fostered by fear of pain and death that leads people to accept cancer therapy. Cancer engenders a particular kind of fear, because it is so insidious. There is never a time when you can say for certain that you are free of it. Cancer follows you like a mental shadow that you have to beat back to remain in the light. Some can live with that better than others. Yet having cancer is not really different from life after a heart attack or stroke, which can also strike again at any time and without warning. Perhaps it is the notion that one is more likely to dispatch you suddenly while the other slowly grinds you down. Perhaps it is the fear of pain and wasting. Any life-threatening condition engenders fear and few come with benign treatment options. But the fear of cancer is particularly unsettling. The imagery of battle with a hideous monster is well entrenched and part of our lives. And the battle must be waged by means that are often destructive. Perhaps cancer frightens us so because it emerges much like a pest that you swat, only to see it rear its ugliness in another corner when you least expect it. The lumps and bumps or abnormal cells in normal places intrude menacingly in a heralded and unwanted blight on what we otherwise consider our exemplary bodies.

Here follows an overview of the prostate cancer therapy options with details to follow in subsequent chapters. All forms of cancer treatment still come with significant side effects because most rely on a narrow margin between destroying cancer cells and injuring normal, healthy cells. Surgery always involves some pain and temporary dysfunction. It also means removal of body tissue, which can produce disfigurement or loss of sexual, urinary, or rectal function. Loss can be minimal and temporary or severe and permanent. Since the change from normal to cancerous prostate cells may not be detectable in its early stages, it is hard to be certain that surgery has eliminated all cancerous tissue. If the surgeon cuts wide to increase the likelihood of cure, the risk of needlessly damaging adjacent tissues is also increased. The area around the prostate gland is chock full of delicate and important structures, so there isn't much leeway. Unfortunately, as with other treatment options, the larger and the more aggressive the cancer, the less the chance that surgery will cure it. Also with increasing age, especially if aging brings on other illness, surgery becomes riskier. For some men, the psychological benefit of believing the tumor is "all out" outweighs other considerations. Surgery is also the best way of sampling areas around the prostate to detect involvement that might otherwise escape detection. Other men will not consider undergoing surgery unless there will be a significant benefit for them, a benefit that outweighs their concerns about the potential for years of incontinence or loss of potency.

Radiation therapy takes advantage of the fact that cancer cells are more sensitive to its effects than normal cells. The radiation beam is a super intense form of light energy. Lead shielding can block X-ray beams, allowing the therapist to limit the damage caused to normal tissues surrounding the prostate. Damage could mean cell death, loss of function, scarring, loss of arterial and nerve supply, or genetic alterations. When radiation damages a cell's genetic material without actually destroying the cell, mutations can occur. This is why radiation can also cause cancer. Both damage to normal tissues and induction of a second malignancy are considerations if you are contemplating having radiation treatment. Once again, age is a factor. It takes years to transform cells to a malignant state, so the second malignancy risk is lower in an older person.

A radiation therapist must gauge tumor containment and design an effective treatment field, without inviting unnecessary tissue and organ damage. There are scanning and new Magnetic Resonance Imaging (MRI) techniques that support this task. However, these aids are not available everywhere, and when push comes to shove, the radiation therapist has to work from probabilities. Tables, based on the biopsy, help predict how likely cancer spread is outside the prostate. Ultimately, every radiation therapy estimate has to be an overestimate, so as not to miss a cancerous area that could remain to grow and cause trouble. If, unbeknownst to the radiation oncologist, the margins of the tumor have extended beyond the radiation field, the treatment will fail. Why not just go for the max? The bladder, intestines, and rectum, which surround and abut the prostate, would then sustain radiation damage. Burning or difficult urination, diarrhea, and food intolerance would be the very unpleasant resulting side effects.

A radiation therapist must also select a dose, that is a final level of radiation to be achieved over a treatment period. Prostate cancer requires a high dose of radiation, and just as with so many forms of cancer treatment, the margin between an effective dose and significant damage to healthy tissue is very narrow. Various new techniques, such as differing radiation beams and fancy shielding, have all been developed to allow for the maximum tumor dose possible. Once again, along with every potential advance comes skepticism, faith, territoriality, grant wars, and the promise of fame and success. Each medical center that has developed a new way to deliver radiation believes in and promotes its approach, sometimes within the profession only, but more often publicly, and on occasion, shamelessly. Not only must you choose whether to have radiation, but you may be faced with machine and technique options that can take you far from your home and family. The added benefits may be marginal, very significant, or simply unknown. Because radiation is given over five to eight weeks' time, such travel can have all sorts of personal and professional ramifications.

Radiation from an X-ray machine, called external beam radiation, is often accompanied by treatment with radioactive seed implants, called brachytherapy. The idea is that the seeds can be placed directly into the prostate gland and can dispense their radiation locally at a high dose with less damage to adjacent tissues than that caused by external beam radiation. The procedure can be done under spinal anesthesia, takes less than an hour, and seems enormously attractive. In fact, in older men especially, brachytherapy is often chosen as the only treatment of prostate cancer thought confined to the gland. It is logical therapy. We would expect it to cure most prostate cancer in this era of early detection. Unfortunately, logic fails us again, and brachytherapy may miss the mark, perhaps because the cancer has spread further than expected. Sometimes, the achieved dose may be more uneven than the seed implanter planned. Radiation in all forms also depends on a target consisting of adequately oxygenated cells. Cancer cells frequently form little viable islands in a bed of dying or dead tissue, rendering the radiation less effective than the dose alone would suggest.

Seeds come at a price. Their placement is often a one-shot deal and irreversible. It's not exactly a shot in the dark, but it's also not completely controlled. In other words, seed implants require a great deal of skill, and are still subject to a certain measure of good or bad luck. Seeds can migrate or escape into the blood stream and potentially lodge in the lungs. They may wind up too close to the urethra, causing inflammation sufficient to interfere with the flow of urine. Generally, seeds cannot be reliably placed in the seminal vesicles, which arise from the prostate and may harbor cancer cells. And once again, the leading seed implant centers have each developed their own approach and techniques. There are differences in the timing of seed placement, the radioactive isotope chosen, permanent or temporary placement, and more. The advantages of one technique over another remain hotly debated, and it may be ten years or more before we know whether one method is really superior to another.

Another treatment possibility is early hormone manipulation. The word "hormone" has some pretty awkward, and occasionally negative, connotations. Men, especially, may falsely construe hormones as substances that primarily affect the lives of women. When girls enter puberty, changes in their behavior are often casually attributed to "hormones." The same goes for women experiencing premenstrual syndrome (PMS) and menopause. The extremes of adolescence are often dismissed as being due to "raging hormones." By contrast, if we men think of male hormones at all, it tends to be in terms of sexual prowess or acne. Or perhaps, hormones are linked to steroids and associated with athletic performance and muscle building.

Both the enormous power and the subtleties of these body chemicals are only dramatically realized when we are deprived of them, as is the case with testosterone reduction in the treatment of prostate cancer. It has long been known that most prostate cancer cells need testosterone to remain viable. If this testosterone is taken away at the tissue level, many cancer cells will die. Unfortunately, genetic mutations, the very same processes that induced the original cancer, cause some cancer cells to become insensitive to the effects of testosterone and to be able to live without it. If this were not the case, testosterone deprivation would be the sole treatment and cure for all prostate cancer.

In the past, testosterone deprivation was accomplished by castration, and it was obviously reserved for cases that failed surgical or radiation treatment. Castration did provide long periods of disease regression. Unfortunately, it did not provide a cure, unless by "cure" we return to the bizarre notion that a man is functionally cured of prostate cancer if he dies from something else. When testosterone is absent, many unpleasant changes ensue, including loss of sexual desire and function, hot flashes and sweats, breast tenderness and growth, thinning of pubic and underarm hair, weight gain, depression, and other mood changes.

Men who are on hormone deprivation treatment are still uncomfortable with the whole concept and may joke about going through male menopause. Often, it is not until the testosterone deprivation ends that the men realize just how affected they were by the changes that took place. A loss of vitality, optimism, and bounce can subvert any man who has prostate cancer and must face both his mortality and the treatment unpleasantnesses. Yet an underlying aura of hormone deprivation can add its own dark flavor to everything else that is happening.

These days, there are a number of reversible, nonsurgical approaches to testosterone deprivation. Two principles are involved. The first is to stimulate the pituitary gland, which gives the signal to produce testosterone to such a degree that supply and ability to meet demand are exhausted. The second principle is to actually block testosterone. Different medications have been developed for each approach: a luteinizing hormone regulating hormone (LHRH), and a number of anti-androgens, androgen being the term for the so called "male" hormones of which testosterone is best known. The LHRH drugs are typically given by injection monthly or at longer intervals. The anti-androgens are taken in pill form, usually several times a day. Depending on the nature of the hormone treatment, the therapy may run a course of months to years. The anti-androgens can actually diminish some of the side effects of LHRH drugs. They also have their own side effects, some so severe as to require discontinuation.

Newer chemotherapeutic and therapeutic antibody approaches will not be considered here because they are mostly still in their experimental infancy, and because clinical trials that use these modalities are still reserved for patients who have relapsed. Similarly, cryosurgery, that is a prostate freezing technique, is generally suggested for older patients who have failed another form of treatment. In the near future, some or all of these treatment choices may become alternatives or adjunct treatment to what is currently available.

No discussion of treatment choices would be complete without paying some attention to diet and lifestyle changes. Granted, this is a fuzzy area, but it has gained legitimacy of late, not only among those who advocate "natural" solutions, but among hardcore scientists as well. For example, it is well established that dietary meat has an impact on testosterone. The incidence of prostate cancer is lowest in countries that have the smallest consumption of meat, and it rises as the level of meat consumption rises. Soy and the lycopene found in tomatoes may inhibit prostate cancer. A trace element, selenium, and estrogen-like compounds found in yams, may do the same. Green vegetables, many noted to be rich in antioxidants, seem to hinder the development of prostate cancer. Some oils and vitamin E may be helpful. Exercise and stress reduction practices may retard the likelihood of cancerous change. While those who engage in evaluating scientific evidence struggle to sort out which of these factors, if any, make a significant difference, each of us has to decide whether changes in diet and lifestyle are warranted in combination with whatever other treatment we choose.

The psychological impact of having choices is enormous. We are ingrained with the idea that the doctor makes a diagnosis and recommends a treatment, period. Most of the time, when choices are presented, the doctor has a strong opinion, hopefully backed by some facts or experience, and this helps the patient choose. With prostate cancer, the choices are many and the knowledge is limited. As a doctor, I used three primary ingredients to arrive at a personal treatment choice. My thought process resembled a mathematical equation in which I tried to take factual knowledge, add in experience, and temper the findings with judgment. My own doctors undoubtedly went through a similar process, but, because the facts are murky and their experience determined by their specialty, their judgment led them to widely differing conclusions. As a doctor-turned-patient, my attempt to follow the equation was also severely compromised. First and foremost, I was really the patient, not the doctor! At the onset, I had very limited and outdated knowledge. As a pediatrician, and even as a pediatric oncologist, I had absolutely no experience with prostate cancer. Children never get prostate cancer. I could not trust my judgment, because it was the prisoner of my emotions. What I wound up doing was concentrating on the acquisition of knowledge. I resurrected approaches to gathering information that dated back to my days as a pediatric hematology/oncology fellow. Using every means at my disposal, I acquired factual knowledge and educated myself as best I could. Lacking my own experience, I created a composite of the experience of others minus their bias, as it was related to me during consultations. Judgment was gleaned from my general approach to medical problems in my pediatric practice. This was the weakest link, and I had to take great pains to maintain a level of doubt about my judgment. I just did my best to apply this inner sense to the decision at hand, hoping my own prejudices and fears would not interfere so much that my judgment would prove faulty. In the end, I had to admit to myself that what I saw as my own judgment was that quality others had referred to as gut feeling. I could only hope that its distillation included a measure of the twenty-five years of accumulated professional decision making that formed my career in medicine.

Another factor in decision making is faith. Faith is a player in all forms of treatment. One needs to have faith in one's doctor and some faith that the chosen treatment represents the best option for you. I believe such faith is earned, not assumed. It accrues not only when your doctor informs and advises you honestly, but when you are able to question, challenge, and actively participate in your treatment and the decisions about your case. Then there is Faith with a capital "F." I happen not to have a great amount of either commodity. Skepticism seems to come more easily to me. But religious or spiritual faith can be a great help to those who possess it and has been shown to improve outcomes and lead to smoother treatment courses. However, relying on faith to the exclusion of medical treatment can be quite hazardous. Medical literature is replete with stories of those who forsook medical care in favor of following beliefs and paid dearly for that decision.

Good statistical outcomes may build faith, but at some point, your own innate faith still becomes the bottom line, because not many a moon will pass before the most rigorous clinician will base a decision on "experience" or "gut feeling" or "judgment," each of which, it turns out, is faith-based! What we call "faith" is simply to adopt as being true a quality that cannot be proven. The most common example given is that of love, which can be inferred from someone's behavior, but can never completely be defined or proven to exist. When someone asks you why you love them, and you answer that it is because of the way they hold your hand, or for their warm smile, or for their honesty, this never really tells the full story. The full story cannot be told, because it resides beyond language in a realm poorly expressed in words. No one has ever seen or held an electron, yet we "know" that it exists. When we get up to go to work each day, we assume the place will still be there from the day before. Much of our faith is built on experience, but we come to a point where we do not act from factual data alone. Some other instinct guides us.

Having faith in one's doctor is a visceral reaction. It need not be complete or blind, and in my case, it was always blocked to a degree by my background and knowledge. As a pediatrician living in an affluent area saturated with other pediatricians, mothers- and fathers-to-be interview me before selecting me as a doctor for their child. During those conversations, I am revealing something intangible about myself, something that may or may not create a bond. The parents-to-be must judge my ability on the basis of the things I say and the manner in which I comport myself. Yet I know that the question they are asking themselves within is, "Can I have a trusting relationship with this doctor?" I have no control over the answer. It is a matter of faith.

In my search, I also conducted interviews of a sort, moving from consultant to consultant, asking questions, developing feelings of more or less trust based on responses I could not rationally measure. I do not readily trust other doctors! To be highly distrustful of one's physicians may hinder the treatment, because a doctor sensing constant scrutiny and suspicion is more apt to screw up. The doctor may not follow his instincts in a misguided attempt to satisfy the patient, and this can lead to trouble. On the other hand, blind trust sometimes leads to a kind of indifference, and the physician may not reach beyond standard approaches or probe the patient's wishes and apprehensions.

In cancer treatment I think trust should be rooted in frankness and humility. So much remains unknown in this field and the stakes are so high that a patient should be able to ask anything of his doctor without feeling he is imposing or stupid. A doctor should encourage discussion of every aspect of the disease and its treatment. In my ideal world, the emotional context of prostate cancer should not remain a taboo between patient and doctor. It should not be shunted to support groups or to other health professionals, unless problems arise that require a higher level of intervention than the treating physician can supply. The discussions surrounding cancer treatment are emotionally loaded and overwhelming. It is easy to misinterpret or forget what has been said. It is both easy and tempting for the doctor to deliver information in time-limited packets, discouraging lengthy and involved questions and responses. I found it useful always to have a listener by my side, my partner or a close relative who knew me, someone I trusted to be sure I heard all that was said and to see that I asked all that was on my mind.

Being on the low side of the trust spectrum, both because of my personality and because of my past experience as a pediatric oncologist, I spent a great deal of time doing my own research, leaving no stone unturned. The process made me anxious, of course, as did the fact of the cancer itself. Furthermore, since "watchful waiting," i.e. doing nothing, is always an option, my family feared I might choose that one and never emerge from the self-imposed research phase. I must admit to being utterly compulsive both in my pursuit of prostate cancer research and in my exhaustive contacts with consultants. This compulsiveness both originated from my anxiety and was its antidote. I remained anxious while I was investigating what I had, perhaps became even a little more anxious in the course of probing treatment options and their consequences. But once I reached my conclusions, I was better able to own them, and I somehow felt less frightened than I had before I began.

Overall, the low-level anxiety that shadowed me for the whole year spanning diagnosis to the end of treatment was largely repressed, although I was told I was more irritable and jumpy. I hid my tension well at work and reserved it for home. It was not until April, during my radiation, that I suffered actual overt episodes of anxiety. The most dramatic of these occurred at a concert when I suddenly developed blurred vision, chest discomfort, and a sense of impending doom. My partner and I stepped outside and I began to feel better. We returned to the concert hall and the symptoms came back. A month later, at the next concert, no sooner did I recall my reaction of the prior month than the light-headedness returned! Then I knew I was a mess. I'll never know whether I would have been better or worse off not doing the extensive research and probing. I believed, on faith, that it was the better approach for me, and so I pursued that path with vigor.

Dealing with so many choices and investigating them so thoroughly proved both painful and exhausting. Yet I felt that in light of the uncertainty surrounding prostate cancer and considering my past training and experience, I owed it to myself to be as educated as possible. In a sense, I was traveling through a maze trying to find the exit. I did eventually emerge, but it was a tortuous process. There were blind alleys, retracing of steps, repetitions and vacillation, all reflected and reported in these pages. In retrospect, I remain pleased that I pursued the effort and made my way through the labyrinth.

Chapter Four

The Path Not Taken

When I first consulted my personal physician, not yet knowing the biopsy results, I was in a state of shock and near hysteria. Imagine if you can, the thoughts of a former pediatric oncologist, one who had begun a career in surgery before switching to pediatrics. I guess all of that could inspire a sense of confidence. In my case, it aroused fear and brought back years of memories. I had witnessed the successes and failures of surgery, both the false claims and the unexpectedly positive results. I had also seen the promise of medical treatment and radiation therapy dashed by complications or a lack of success. I had been party to my own oncology patients' fates, those who should have survived their cancer but did not, as well those who were thought doomed but somehow survived. My pessimism was not groundless, but it was exaggerated as a consequence of apprehension and past experiences. I had a healthy respect for the vagaries of cancer and knowledge of how little we can control the outcomes.

So when my physician assured me I was not about to die from this cancer, I was not entirely mollified. Actually, I barely heard him, and I didn't believe what he was saying. When I asked him what he would do in my situation, he said he would probably choose surgery, more for psychological reasons than for coldly rational ones. He was inclined to hope that they could "get it all out." Surgery lures us with its promise of total excision of the tumor, a temptation that is hard to resist. Indeed, when surgery removes all malignant tissue along with the gland from which the cancer arose, the apparent cure rate is excellent. Nothing can quite replace taking out all cancerous tissue and what ever else has the potential to become cancerous. Surgery seems so clean and direct. In the face of a promise of successful surgery, wouldn't any reasonable person take a chance on the side effects and go for the possibility of cure?

Yet I was predisposed to avoid surgery in general and this surgery in particular. This was my own bias speaking. It is undisputed that surgery can cure small prostate cancers. What remains an open question is whether other forms of treatment can perform as well with a lower complication rate. Anyway, mine was not a small tumor. The whole gland was involved. It happens that I am quite frightened of having surgery, especially surgery involving general anesthesia. Quite a confession for a doctor! There is a known constellation of fear of dying, fear of flying, and fear of anesthesia. I happen to be one of those so afflicted. I do go on airplane flights despite some misgivings about the whole thing. I have had hernia surgery, albeit performed under local anesthesia (but accompanied by sedation so heavy I might as well have had a general). I have gone through postoperative pain and experienced both its discomfort and the eventual dissipation of that discomfort. At that time, I thought "I can do this again if I have to." But when actually confronted with the prospect of having surgery again, I was petrified.

Why fear surgery or anesthesia? We rely on an expectation of continuing life, moment-to-moment, day-to-day, year-to-year, despite the certainty of death and those nightly news reminders that human destruction can approximate that of the smallest insect. We voluntarily submit to sleep with the expectation that we will wake up. We willingly encase ourselves in aluminum shells that take us to 40,000 feet into the air and assume that we will land safe and sound. Those who are comfortable with anesthesia go under confident they will emerge as conscious and aware as they were before. These expectations are perfectly reasonable, based on demonstrated safety and reproducibility.

Being leery of surgery, my first reaction to the MRI diagnosis of cancer was that I hoped the tumor could be eradicated by some form of radiation, thus allowing me to avoid the knife. Little did I imagine that the tumor would be so large and widespread that surgery might not even be suggested as the best option. As my doctor was speaking, I remembered my own patients asking me, "So what would you do if you were in my place?" I always reminded them that I was not. Advice given in theory may deviate from what is done when the situation becomes a personal reality. Given the same set of facts, various doctors may come to different conclusions, especially when those facts contain a degree of uncertainty. But no one, especially not an "objective" doctor, can step into the shoes of someone who is ill or injured. We are too complex and our needs and expectations are too varied to offer simple solutions that apply to every person. In my conversations with other men, I encountered some for whom life without sex was not worth living. An equal number were antsy about the thought of being "zapped" by radiation. It should come as no surprise to those for whom Hiroshima, Chernobyl, and other disasters have emotional immediacy, that radiation is dangerous. Women radiated for acne have developed breast cancer later in life. Watches with radium numerals on their faces have been shown to cause cancer. Radiation damage from the sun has resulted in an upsurge of skin cancer. Everyone knows that radiation is not good for you. It burns and genetically injures everything in the path of its beam.

I met men who could not stand the notion that any viable tumor cells, which could have been removed by surgery, might be left in the body, even if they were treated with radiation doses that should kill all cancer cells. Some men were comfortable with a degree of uncertainty, while others were intent on guarantees, or at least the hope that a surgeon could report that the cancer appeared to be gone after surgery. Nothing can quite beat the confidence instilled by a postoperative report that the surgical margins were clear and there was no evidence of residual tumor. Yet we know that at least some of these patients will relapse, and this information can certainly temper a patient's enthusiasm for prostate surgery.

For some like me, surgery is particularly frightening because it seems so definitive in the negative sense. That which is removed cannot be restored. A notable exception is reconstructive, or plastic, surgery, not a consideration where the prostate gland is concerned. What is taken out does not recover function because it is permanently gone, never again to be part of your body. If an excess of healthy tissue has been removed, something has been sacrificed to seek a cure, and it is lost for good. This point is important because adequate tumor surgery must provide those tumor-free margins where microscopic examination of the removed tumor confirms a cancer-free zone of normal tissue. Lacking tumor-free margins, surgery may prove a failure, or radiation treatment may also be needed on top of the surgery to achieve the potential for a cure that eluded the surgeon. The hooker is that even if margins appear cancer-free under the microscope, there is no guarantee that the cancerous process has not already spread beyond those margins to cells that still look normal. This explains why patients who are found to have free tumor margins both to the naked eye and under the microscope nevertheless can and do relapse.

The surgical path has become the so-called "gold standard" against which other forms of treatment are measured. To digress for a moment, in the past, the field of medicine was neatly divided into two realms, that of the surgeon and that of the medical physician. Some medical schools still bear this distinction, physicians and surgeons. In many countries, surgeons are still known as Mister while medical physicians are called Doctor. Especially in the preantibiotic and prechemotherapy eras, the treatment of illnesses was typically relegated to one of these realms; surgeons dealt with appendicitis, malformations, cancer, and abscesses and medical doctors treated heart disease, stroke, and diabetes. Subsequently, overlap crept in with the consequence that one group became primary and the other secondary, acting as consultants. Thus a patient with lung cancer would have surgery, and if the patient developed a fever, the surgeon would call in an internist or infectious disease medical specialist as a consultant. Conversely, if a cancer patient developed an abscess or needed a tube replaced, a surgeon would be called in as a consultant and would perform the procedure. More recently, the lines of separation have further been blurred as new specialties have arisen that straddle the fields. Radiologists now put tubes and stents in a variety of locations in the field of Invasive Radiology.

In the past, surgery was the initial attack launched on all solid tumor malignancies like breast and prostate cancer. This is why surgery has historically been the first treatment against prostate cancer. As the gold standard, still held to be inherently superior to other forms of therapy, surgery continues to be the preferred treatment option for young, otherwise healthy men, whose tumors are considered confined to the gland. This path of referral colors the decision-making process, and places a degree of pressure on patients to accept the standard practice. This means the general physician or internist who detects a prostate problem is likely to refer the patient to a urologist, both for biopsy and for The Decision. To be fair, most urologists will suggest that their patients also speak with a radiation therapist. But urology, being a surgical subspecialty, breeds urologists who, of course, are surgeons and lean toward the surgical approach. Until relatively recently, urologists dominated the treatment of prostate cancer and accounted for most of the experts in the field. The goal of surgery has remained largely unchanged, that is to cut out the tumor, which in essence means removing the prostate gland plus some surrounding tissue. In meeting this primary goal, there has been little recent innovation in surgical technique. Surgical progress has been directed primarily at making a difficult operation easier, reducing the negative consequences of the surgery, and making it possible to perform the operation on older and sicker people. Overall, however, the success of surgery has not been that great. Specialists developing alternative forms of treatment have had to confront the monolith of surgery and the preconceived notion that it remains the best way to proceed for anyone who can tolerate it, provided there is no evidence of spread beyond the gland. It is very hard to undermine a gold standard.

The surgery being discussed here is termed radical prostatectomy. The word "radical" is frightening and conjures up its equivalent in women, radical mastectomy, in which the whole breast, together with lymph nodes and muscle, are removed. Radical prostatectomy is a bit less radical. Some lymph nodes are sampled for the presence of tumor as the surgeon proceeds toward the gland itself. Sampling lymph nodes is a good practice because surgery alone cannot cure the patient if the tumor has spread to the lymph nodes.

It is now possible to watch surgery on television, an entertainment of sorts, so the general public is no longer spared the gory details. A scalpel is used to make a skin incision. The cut is typically vertical, from above the navel to the pubic area. To reach the prostate, the surgeon combines blunt (tearing) with sharp (cutting) dissection. The surgeon tries to take advantage of the natural separation between layers of fat, muscle, and organs, known as tissue planes. The goal is both to expose the prostate and minimize actual trauma to the tissues. On the other hand, an old mentor of mine said, in effect, you never want a plastic surgeon doing tumor surgery. Any cosmetic considerations need to remain in the background, at least until the tumor is excised as completely as possible. Electrocautery is used both to seal off bleeding blood vessels and to carry out sharp dissection. The surgeon holds a pencil-like instrument and works a pedal on the floor to control the current. You might hear the hiss on television, but you also get to experience the smell of burning flesh if you happen to find yourself in the operating room.

Removal of the entire prostate gland deserves the added "radical" because the surrounding structures, to some degree, must be damaged. Since the prostate wraps around the urethra, from which urine flows out of the bladder, the urethra must be cut and separated in order to remove the gland. Because the tumor may invade the seminal vesicles, which produce semen, these must be removed, potentially damaging the nerves that provide sensation and erections. During the past years nerve-sparing techniques have been developed and are largely successful, provided the surgeon believes potential spread to that area low. The surgeon's judgment about the nerves is based on the biopsy findings corroborated by inspection at the time of surgery. If there is tumor near the nerves, it can spread alongside their path. The surgeon must avoid injury to the rectum or bladder while still removing all visible tumor. The operation entails a fair amount of blood loss, so the patient can, and generally does, donate his own blood in advance for subsequent transfusion. The blood donation typically begins six weeks before surgery, providing plenty of time during which you are free to anticipate and worry about the operation.

It must seem strange to walk into the blood bank while you are feeling well, donate blood, spend weeks building yourself up from at least some degree of anemia, do the whole thing again, preparing to be bled during surgery that has no immediacy for you while you are in the auto-donation process. People often ask why a relative cannot donate the blood so that you can get on with the surgery before you have to worry too much about it. Well it turns out that random blood, that is blood obtained from unrelated donors, is statistically safer than designated units donated by a family member. This curious fact stems from the finding that relatives are apt to conceal illnesses they may not wish to reveal to other kin. Furthermore, the donation, storage, and administration process runs a risk of errors. The wrong person may receive a designated unit. Or the unit may be contaminated in the course of processing.

In experienced hands, the radical prostatectomy procedure takes approximately three hours, and the postoperative course involves about five days in the hospital. Drains are placed in cavities created by surgery, and the absence of the prostate gland creates just such a cavity. Until the body has filled in what is missing, bleeding, fluid accumulation, and infection may arise. A drain is therefore left in the pelvic cavity and is typically removed just before discharge. I have been told that taking out this drain really hurts. Deep tissue pain and incision pain are much easier to control. Patient-controlled analgesia (PCA) is currently in fashion, and thankfully so. A defined amount of narcotic, usually morphine, is added to your IV and runs through a machine that can be programmed to deliver the drug in restricted amounts and at preprogrammed time intervals. So, if you need to walk to the bathroom, you can time the excursion and give yourself a dose of morphine just a few minutes before you go. Despite all the cutting and probing, I have heard radical prostatectomy patients describe their postoperative pain as being quite tolerable.

Doctors have learned that in the past, we failed to achieve adequate pain control, even when it was technically possible. Justification offered for under-treatment included fear of masking symptoms that could indicate a serious surgical problem. This seems generally to be a nonissue. Another objection arose from fear of narcotic addiction, once again a false concern. People taking narcotics short-term for pain control do not become junkies. Those medicines make you feel so weird you just can't wait to stop. This is especially true when a hallucination has you imagining birds in your room or bugs crawling up your legs. It is not necessary to have the added indignity of Demerol injections when PCA using very small amounts of morphine does the job just fine.

As the pain subsides, and the relief of being past the surgery sinks in, the urine catheter becomes the patient's next issue. Because the urethra is severed, all patients must have an indwelling catheter at least two to three weeks after the surgery. The catheter provides a conduit for urine flow, and it also allows the urethral tissue to heal around it. The normal plumbing is arranged such that there are a couple of places where the tissues form a kind of sling that can constrict or relax, allowing us to control the flow of our urine. These anatomic sphincters are lost in the surgical procedure. The surgeon has to reconstruct a urinary sphincter, a formidable challenge. The surgeon also has to navigate the little nerves that allow for sexual function, assuming the patient's cancer is situated where it can be removed while those nerves are spared. Depending on the patient's age, the degree to which he had strong sexual functions before the surgery, and whether or not he has taken hormones, a patient may recover a ranging degree of sexual function. After the urine catheter is removed, incontinence can last days to months as can loss of sexual function; either erection or orgasm could be impaired. There is no guarantee that either will return to the preoperative state: some side effects may be permanent, and ejaculates are usually dry.

So why not just have radiation and reserve surgery for later if relapse occurs? By comparison, radiation seems so much less invasive, and it is, but this is not to say that is not without its own set of complications. If radiation fails, subsequent surgery is even more difficult, because the tissues are scarred much as though they had been burned, and the normal tissue planes of dissection may be matted together or obliterated entirely. While normal tissues are not removed as with surgery, they are injured by the radiation, so bladder and bowel problems can arise, resulting in chronic urinary difficulty or diarrhea and rectal bleeding. Radiation can make you feel tired and weak. In contrast to surgery, where things tend to slowly improve after the initial insult, the complications of radiation can sneak up on you. Some worsen as the years pass. Finally, perhaps the most dreaded complication could be a second malignancy, usually of the bladder or bowel. The same radiation that cures cancer can cause cancer, because it attacks our genes and produces mutations. Both the potential for success and the risk of complications must be weighed, for surgery as well as for radiation.

Following surgery, complete recovery leading to return to work and full activity typically takes two months or more. By contrast, those receiving radiation may continue to work throughout, or experience brief periods of fatigue towards the end of the treatment course. Depending on the pathology findings, some surgical patients may need postoperative radiation anyway, in which case the complications may become additive. I talked to some people who had radical prostatectomy and sailed through the whole thing, some who had experienced complications, and others who had uncertain or incomplete return of continence and sexual function. I encountered a deep commitment to the procedure amongst those who had had it done. What I came to understand was that few people would go through this kind of surgery, suffer its complications, receive a good prognosis (surgeons tend to be optimists), and then turn around and say it wasn't worth it. Such a conclusion might even jinx the outcome. There was a need, I felt, for those who had surgery to believe it had been entirely successful, the right decision, and worthwhile. In a sense, surgery is not for doubters.

If one can risk a generalization, surgeons themselves, both by temperament and by training, tend not to be doubters. Confidence seems to be a necessary requirement for the surgeon, and it is hard to imagine a patient who would willingly consent to have surgery performed by a physician who harbors self-doubt! Can you imagine a surgeon saying that he thought he might be able to accomplish something for you, but wasn't really sure and didn't have all that much experience with cases like yours, but what the heck, how about we give it a try? Would you want this person to cut on you?

Unfortunately, the first cousin of this very quality of confidence is arrogance, and the dividing line may be a fine one indeed. This is not said as criticism or an unfair generalization, put rather to make a positive point. A measure of arrogance becomes an attribute for surgeons. We must recognize that a surgeon's charge is to physically disassemble, then repair or rebuild the human body, an undertaking that lends itself to high drama and tension as well as to impressive and immediate gratification. Furthermore, the action is a quick and definitive fix, human carpentry, in and out, done. Truly, here appears to be God's work in man's hands. In fact, surgeons who are admired for their technical skill by colleagues are often described as having good hands, revered for their manual ability as though some superhuman talent had been bestowed upon them.

To fully appreciate the emotional power of surgery, sports and military analogies are somewhat appropriate. Teams and soldiers battle it out, even against superior forces. There are underdogs who struggle to overcome daunting odds. Like gladiators, surgeons may find themselves cast into the arena against tumors having the ferocity of lions. They play to the last out, even if they are losing. Long hours in the operating room call to mind marathons. Tense moments resemble tightrope walking at the circus. The champions of surgery, like sports heroes may attain both fame and the unswerving admiration of fans, be they staff, fellow physicians, or patients. If they are in the "big leagues," typically university medical centers, they may command large salaries, although, sad to say, sports still seem to be accorded far greater value than either surgery or medicine!

Now, you want your surgeon to have both good hands and a good head, because judgment and decisiveness under time pressure accompanies every surgical decision. With decisiveness, swift and sure judgment, and good hands, may come a certain impatience. To cut is to know what must be done. Many surgeons want to get it done, by temperament as well as by conviction. As a consequence, there may be a tendency for surgeons to yield only slowly to alternative treatment possibilities. It should come as no surprise that surgeons would need overwhelming proof of success before recommending something other than removal of the gland containing the cancer. And while doctors with a more medical orientation certainly include surgery in their treatment armamentarium, surgeons are often disinterested, or even uninvolved, in the details of nonsurgical patient management.

I recall a departmental policy that was in effect during my pediatric training. Every pediatric surgical patient admitted to the ward had to be seen by the pediatric resident, and daily rounds and chart reviews were conducted on these children. Our Chief felt that pediatric surgery was just another subspecialty of pediatrics, just like pediatric cardiology, although the training followed another pathway. While we residents had little interest in surgical detail, we had to be involved from beginning to end. Although the surgeons may have been less interested in the nonsurgical problems of their patients, they could not entirely escape them. By means of enforced contact, surgical and medical doctors-in-training were required to work together and learn from each other. The same relationship was present during my oncology training when the specialties met at a Tumor Board to discuss cases. I would have liked to benefit from such cross-fertilization among specialties.

I had heard from my urologist that the prostate surgeon at the medical center in my region was more open to nonsurgical treatment than your average surgeon, and I found this comforting, given my prejudices. Since I was leaning against surgery anyway,

I thought I might find a balanced opinion—balanced, of course, meaning being in agreement with my own thoughts on the matter. So I shamelessly used connections to get an early appointment. We all know that a doctor-turned-patient should be treated the same as a mister-patient, but this clearly is not the case, for which I was thankful. MRI in hand, I suffered the indignities of patient registration and elevators crowded with doctors and patients, and went up to the urology clinical suites. Since pediatric private practice tends to be informal, I do not wear a white coat in my own daily doctoring work. But here at the university medical center, rank and stature were in the air. There is nothing smaller and more vulnerable than a patient with a life-threatening illness seeking help from the elevated starched white coats. The faculty clinic building and the urology suite formed an imposing unit, its rather narrow waiting room offering a bay view to rival that of any restaurant atop an office building. I didn't feel like the powerful doctor anymore.

My encounter with the university medical center's expert prostate surgeon was pleasant and informative. We chatted about common acquaintances and reminisced about shared past experiences. He examined me. This was beginning to feel like a routine. He went over the data, the extent of my disease, my MRI. When all was said and done, he pronounced me a good candidate for surgery and stated his belief that my tumor might well still be contained in the gland. However, considering the location, extent, and aggressiveness of the tumor, nerve sparing was not an option. Everything would have to go. I was not prepared for this. But there it was, his opinion, the honest assessment and judgment of a recognized world expert, someone not to be discounted. Here was a master prostate surgeon telling me that he thought I could be cured in his hands, the justification being his experience. How was I to receive this assessment with equanimity? Our discussion deviated to the details of surgery, the anesthesia, the technique, and the complications. He made it all sound relatively easy and painted a very encouraging long-term picture, one suggesting a low rate of enduring complications in his hands. Even my fear of general anesthesia was overcome. I could have a spinal. Throughout our discussion, the word "cure" seemed to dangle in front of me, although it was never explicitly stated.

Nevertheless, despite all the optimism, I knew these complications could be very nasty. When you open books for the laymen that describe treatment options, the surgery section invariably points out the two complications that stand out like no others: incontinence and impotence. By comparison, the more basic margin failures seem to take up less space and receive less attention. Pages are devoted to these complications and methods to counter them. Between the two issues, impotence seems to carry the greater emotional punch. I do not know whether the question has been studied scientifically, but I suspect that this is a greater issue for the men so affected than it is for their sexual partners. Our very self-esteem seems linked to the ability of the organ in question to rise to the occasion. The very word "performance" says it all.

Books list a collection of contraptions and devices to assist sexual performance, devices that would be the envy of someone writing a medieval torture manual. Not that the implements necessarily cause pain. They just have that appearance when diagrammed. There are vacuum devices, rods that provide permanent erections, requiring yet other maneuvers to re-create the normal, unaroused state. There are procedures to self-inject the penis or instill stimulating substances into the urethra. And, of course, there is the V drug, advertised and popularized by a former presidential candidate and the brunt of a never-ending series of jokes, some actually quite funny. This is not to belittle the pleasure associated with a properly functioning erect penis. It simply emphasizes the less than benign consequences of non-nerve-sparing prostate surgery. Incontinence also is onerous. Urine smells and is associated with a lack of cleanliness or senility. For those who expect to recover continence but do not, the consequences of surgery can be even more upsetting. Once again there are a variety of surgical solutions to this surgical complication, consisting of indwelling inflatable balloons and other similar devices.

Reacting to the hope dangled before me, I blurted out that the last thing I wanted was to go through the trauma of surgery only to emerge with the finding that margins were positive for tumor requiring radiation on top of the surgery. There was new data emerging to show that postsurgical radiation could handle at least one positive margin, one little area where tumor penetrated the prostate capsule, but this could heap complications on top of complications and still prove ineffectual. As our time drew to a close, I asked for surgical outcome data in patients like me, those with my stage, my Gleason score, my PSA, and my MRI. The surgical consultant said he would get back to me within a few days by email once he had reviewed his database. Our interview ended with me in no way reassured and doubting my ability to choose what treatment would be best for me. While I didn't want surgery, I very much felt the pressure to yield to its offer of hope and permanent cure.

A few days later, I received a crisp email saying that it would take longer than expected to retrieve the outcome data I had requested, and, in thinking further about my case, perhaps it would be better to have radiation. Anyway, the email reported new innovative surgical techniques were being developed for those who relapse after radiation. Sure enough, very recently, advertisements have appeared in the local newspaper recruiting relapsed patients into a study to evaluate these techniques. When this down-the-line option was laid at my doorstep, I felt that the aura of competitive disagreement between prostate specialists was palpable. There was a barely disguised implication that I was pretty much bound to relapse after radiation. I already knew that surgery after radiation comes at a great price, with higher rates of complications, especially more incontinence. Or was I reading more into his words than I should?

The tone of the email somehow made me feel that it was my lack of enthusiasm, my doubting the surgeon's evaluation and pronouncements, not simply the hard facts of my case, which led to my dismissal as a good candidate for surgery. I was also left with the nagging question of whether my own fear and procrastination were responsible for this situation. Even though I knew better, even though I knew prostate cancer extends slowly, even though I knew that this cancer had been present for years, even though none of my doctors had insisted on earlier biopsy, I felt that I had somehow let them down because of cowardice. Anxiety and vulnerability play bad tricks on the mind.

I also felt partially relieved that the surgical door seemingly had been closed more by circumstances than by a simple choice of mine. Nevertheless, about ten minutes after making the decision to skip surgery, doubts crept into my thinking. Was it a mistake motivated by simple fear? Would I regret it later when surgery was no longer an option? The closing of a therapeutic door always leads to some measure of "what if" self-doubt, especially if there are wrinkles in the alternative treatment that has been chosen. I still wonder about surgery. How would it have been for me? What if, after surgery had been done, margins had been clear, and complications had not occurred? What if sexual function had been permanently lost, and I had to rely on medications for sexual activity? Would that have been a fair trade-off for a greater certainty of cure? Would I have felt a greater certainty of cure? Is there objectively a greater certainty of cure? Many people make such decisions easily and do not look back at the wisdom of their choice. Others may be plagued by both their choice and by living with its consequences. Unfortunately, I found myself in the latter camp, especially while I was receiving treatment and experiencing side effects. For me, and I suspect for others, there had never been a choice like this one, not professionally, not in my personal life. I had not taken the well-intentioned advice of one of the foremost urologists in prostate cancer treatment. Who was I to turn this advice aside? And this was only the beginning, my first consultation to lay out the course of treatment. I left surgery behind as a treatment option, but it continued to rear its head long afterward. Other consultants mentioned surgery, and it remained a never-ending subject of discussion when I talked with nonmedical folk who just assumed it was *the* treatment for prostate cancer.

I should stress that I am not trying to dissuade anyone from having surgery, but rather telling this part of the story to reveal the anguish and self-doubt that accompanied my first decision of major consequence. Others may experience the same kind of torment over different aspects of this journey. I am also attempting to illustrate how past experience, fear, and prejudice can weigh in heavily and disrupt objectivity. I still believe I made the correct decision for myself. By this, I mean the whole of myself, not just the diseased part of myself. I recognize well that it was much more than a decision based on cold medical fact. I will always have to live with this knowledge and accept its consequences, whatever they may turn out to be.

Chapter Five

Talking to Everyone

It is challenging to try to capture the full impact of the lengthy phase of research and consultations that followed my diagnosis. It reaches back to the time immediately following my receipt of MRI results, when I first made phone contact with the doctor in Seattle who would eventually do my implant. It both precedes and follows my consultation with the university-based prostate surgeon. It reflects a period of time when all approaches, all kinds of treatment, all the places offering treatment, were being considered, weighed in my mind, compared one against the other. Even surgery, which I thought I had dismissed early in the game, continued to be a part of the mental mix, albeit pretty far down the list. Nothing was completely eliminated until I took steps that precluded others namely, lying down to receive radiation. Even the beginning of treatment did not eliminate choices and months ensued during which my grinding exploration of prostate cancer treatment options persisted and dominated my life. It is not important to review this period with absolute chrono-logical accuracy. What matters is to capture the flavor of four con-verging factors. First, my own urologist and the first radiation oncologist I saw both told me I could take my time arriving at a therapy decision. The progression of prostate cancer is slow, they said, and a few more weeks make no difference whatsoever. Second, I tend to have a hard time making important personal decisions that involve choices or advance planning. Third, because of my training and experience in pediatric oncology, I had the ability to do fairly extensive research. Fourth, I didn't trust any-one else to do this research for me. The result was a period of months, during which I read articles written for the lay public, pored over medical journals, spent hours on the computer, and pursued person-to-person, telephone, and email consultations worldwide.

Some of my encounters were serendipitous. One day, I was in the hospital medical library, and I decided to review journals by picking up and perusing each current volume on the shelf that might contain an applicable article. There were general journals, such as *The Journal of the American Medical Association* (JAMA), *The Lancet, The British Medical Journal, The New England Journal of Medicine,* science journals, such as *Nature* and *Scientific American,* and specialty journals such as *Urology* and *The Journal of Urology.* I looked through each table of contents, a very ineffi-cient way to obtain pointed information. I also looked at the Letters to the Editor sections, because here, at the fringes of each journal, places reminiscent of predallas (the lower margins of some Renaissance paintings), one often finds interesting and novel approaches to problems.

I was coming up empty handed in the library, when I suddenly saw the cover of a nursing journal featuring a lead article on seed implantation for prostate cancer. It was here that I encountered my first detailed introduction to seeds, and, because it was a nursing journal, I was able to read about the different varieties, techniques, and problems surrounding this procedure in relatively straightforward, simple language. As I read the article with care, I was both intrigued and encouraged by what seemed to be a logical and slick approach to this cancer, one that was relatively less invasive than surgery. The article's virtue also proved to be its downfall. Because its audience was neither that of the decision-making clinician nor that of the research physician, the article lacked an informative review of outcome data. Some of my initial enthusiasm would subsequently be doused by articles from surgical and radiation therapy disciplines.

A colleague handed me more information about seeds in an unlikely source. This was an article in a business magazine detailing the diagnosis, decision-making process, and treatment of a Silicon Valley executive. Here, too, I learned more about seed implants as well as the group of doctors in Seattle that specialized in prostate seeding. The article was well written and captured the flavor of the divergence of opinions surrounding this cancer. It provided validation of the personal nature of prostate cancer decision making, delivered by someone from the business world, a man presumably familiar with making definitive decisions. As I pored over these and other papers, I began to accumulate material, seeking out so-called review articles, in which experts in the field cover broad subjects for a general medical readership. From the various biases and opposing convictions,

I could tell this was destined to be a long and confusing process. There were few uniformly accepted paths. Even when it came to seemingly simple manners, such as what is a normal PSA and when is a biopsy needed, informed opinions varied widely. How would I ever sort this out, especially given the injection of my own fears and prejudices?

Other avenues exist for the exchange of information. In my own case, I did not want to join a support group. I do not like to participate in scheduled meetings devoted to a shared dilemma, listening to the problems of others. I now wanted to be the center of attention. I was also afraid I might become doctor to the group, someone that lay members turned to, at a time when I needed friendship and talk focused on my own concerns. This may have been an unfounded fear, but it determined my behavior anyway. The Internet provides chat rooms, but I found that anonymous stories frequently tended to be horror accounts, which could not properly be evaluated without knowing the source. They therefore carried the hazard of being more frightening than reassuring. I did not explore this avenue further. As a doctor, what I found most useful were my conversations with other doctors who had been through prostate cancer treatment, and I spoke with many of those. In fact, one of my pediatric colleagues and I thought about starting a doctor's cancer support group within our own hospital's medical staff, but we rejected the idea precisely because doctors who knew each other would likely not be forthright and revealing in an open forum.

I chose a different route. Somewhat obsessively, I began to call people. By the time it was all over, I had contacted about thirty experts or fellow patients. This is not a straightforward story to tell because it evolved in multiple ways. One call often led to another. Others derived from articles I read. Some were fishing expeditions. Some occurred by accident, a chance meeting, the advice of a friend. My own obsession with making the best choice was the driving engine. Many people would do just fine leaving the decisions to a trusted physician, and others would self-impose some limit on opinions sought. But my story serves to illustrate just how convoluted a path can be if you let it go wherever it takes you.

It is peculiar that one can read about innovations in journals, or more often these days in the newspapers and magazines, long before it is appropriate to avail oneself of them. It used to be the case that advances were reported in medical journals exclusively, then evaluated, challenged, and reproduced or abandoned after years of further study. But many scientists who engage in research have discovered the glory of headlines. As a consequence, what appears in popular publications when it is "discovered" sometimes disappears years later when it does not amount to anything. In my own practice, I am often confronted with ideas that are not yet medically proven, cures that emerge from out of the blue, fashionable material downloaded from the Net. It is hard enough to keep up with new information contained in medical journals, and even there, much turns out to be a flash in the pan. Imagine what it is like to add in the stuff on talk shows, in the lay press, and on TV specials. The dissemination of preliminary findings is not all bad, but when it raises false hopes it becomes medically insincere.

Some of my phone contacts also urged me to get a second opinion on the biopsy, since one person's Gleason 7 might be another's 6 or 8. One of the leading prostate pathologists worked in the Midwest. It happens we had overlapped in training some twenty years before, but we did not know each other. I placed the call, fully expecting to speak to a secretary or a pathology fellow. I was quite surprised when he answered the phone himself as though I had just called him at home. This master pathologist was generous both with his time and his advice. No need for a second opinion, he said, the pathology at the institution where I had my biopsy was excellent. But, he asked me, would I care for his clinical opinion? Here was a turn! Of course, I said, knowing that pathologists don't treat living patients. In fact, I think it fair to say that most pathologists would shy away from expressing a clinical opinion. But this guy knew his way around prostate cancer. His opinion was not to be discounted. "Get yourself an excellent surgeon," he said. He was both emphatic and impassioned on the subject. Pandora's box opened again!

Perhaps sensing my plodding pace and seeming procrastination, he emphasized that there was absolutely no justification for "watchful waiting." To my way of thinking, the whole concept seems a misnomer anyway. Virtually all cancer patients practice watchful waiting in one form or another after exposing their malignancy to some kind of treatment or lifestyle change ranging from least to most invasive. Only the very aged or the very stubborn do absolutely nothing. Whatever intervention is chosen, there inevitably follows a period of watchful waiting, typically years, when we wait to see whether the cancer progresses or returns. This pathologist emphasized that the natural growth of prostate cancer is slow, but relentless. Eventually the nature of the cancer changes and it becomes aggressive and spreads quickly.

As a "young person," I would experience this fate at an earlier age if I did not do something to counter the cancer's presence and growth. Of course one could find some reports that held that prostate cancer could be left alone without much change in overall statistical outcome, but most experts in this country roundly criticized such conclusions. So, the only issue in this pathologist's mind was how soon I should undergo surgery.

There followed a very strong pitch for removal of the primary tumor and a lymph node biopsy, supported by his belief as a pathologist in examining tissue and proper staging. He told me about data that suggested good outcomes after radical prostatectomy, even in patients with positive surgical margins or a micropositive lymph node, provided that radiation followed the surgery. He even offered and subsequently sent me a computerized comparison of the long-term outcome of surgery versus radiation for my stage and Gleason score, which showed an advantage for surgery.

The pathologist gave me a personalized computer print-out, one based on a sophisticated prostate cancer prognosis model, virtually indicating I would be a fool not to have surgery. Data was missing, however, on external beam radiation plus seeds. Such projections can be helpful but they can also be misleading. Individual variation and details not incorporated into the database do not figure in the calculation, although they may have real-life implications that have yet to be defined by the statisticians. In any case, when this influential expert heard the name of my potential radiation therapist, he backed off a bit, saying he trusted him, and I might do just as well with radiation if I really was not considering surgery. He apparently saw prostate cancer as an anatomic manifestation of evil in the world and told me to, "Fight the monster." He too wished me good luck. So many of the people I consulted ended their recommendations with the words "good luck."

Some time later, speaking with a prostate oncologist in Seattle, I had a similar experience. Showing some bias, I thought, she stressed that seeds were not as benign as portrayed, and that she'd seen many failures and complications with implants. She was located at a university medical center in Seattle, home to one of the leading prostate surgeons, and admittedly was a surgery proponent, telling me that it paid to de-bulk the tumor, even if additional treatment had to be given subsequently. De-bulking is a term coined for partial, therefore incomplete, surgical removal of cancer. I remained unconvinced, especially in the face of contrary opinions from radiation therapists. But these two strong opinions favoring surgery rattled me again. Here were two leaders in the field both telling me things I did not want to hear. I now had to face the possibility that I had made up my mind in advance and was simply not listening to reason.

When I saw the local university-based radiation oncologist, a very different point of view emerged. For my degree of tumor involvement, his data strongly implied that radiation and seeds offered long-term cure rates comparable to surgery at a comparatively lower risk of complications. This consultation was not a quickie visit or phone call, but included a protracted discussion with an extensive review of the literature. Of course, the literature itself is subject to interpretation and fraught with the possibility of bias. Even with my level of medical sophistication, reviewing and evaluating all the papers that he presented to me would have required time and expertise that I lacked. Nevertheless, his analysis was impressive. He was impressive. I left his office leaning toward radiation, but still troubled by the equally strong opposing opinions of other experts.

Some days later, I was walking from my office to a neighborhood café when I unexpectedly ran into the father of a former patient. He was also a physician and had moved out of the area to head a research division in a pharmaceutical company, so I was surprised to see him. We chatted about his family and mine and then I told him about my problem. It turned out that he had had to find a urologist for his father and had been working with a university-based doctor in Pennsylvania whom he thought both straightforward and well-informed about prostate cancer. I called this referral a number of times, and he turned out to be exactly as advertised—blunt, positive, and honest.

Why do I say, honest? Anyone invested in a treatment modality has a measure of bias, which, no matter how subtle, my training helps me detect readily. This physician, a urologist, was a surgeon, but not an advocate of surgery for everybody, and was not one for simply following the latest vogue. In his opinion, surgery alone had a low chance of success in cases such as mine. He advised radiation, saying he doubted it would cure me, but that I would probably have ten, maybe fifteen disease-free years after which, who knows.

Why was it encouraging to be told I would have a good disease-free interval and then relapse? Depending on your perspective, ten to fifteen years may sound short or long. But this was the first person to remind me that prostate cancer was an illness of possibilities, that the future was promising, that many who should have done poorly had lived with this illness for years longer than expected. He also was the first urologist, the first surgeon, to agree with my assessment that surgery was not necessarily the best answer to this problem, and that the "success" of the surgical approach was overrated. In fact, it was his opinion that no one, and certainly not he, really understood prostate cancer at all. I was now more committed to a radiation path, but was still faced with the type of radiation to be delivered, the location of the treatment, and the question of radiation alone or radiation plus implants.

I encountered two new choices, one regional and one distant. The regional route was familiar: the university medical center where I had studied and first worked as a pediatric oncologist. The second route was to the East Coast. On the regional side, I did not want to omit speaking with people with whom I had actually worked, albeit almost twenty years ago. Some were doctors with whom I had little contact. Others, especially the pediatric radiation therapist, were people with whom I had a close working relationship, sometimes testy, sometimes elating, sometimes depressing, but a professional history nevertheless. During my years in pediatric oncology, the radiation therapy suite was located at the main hospital, separate from the children's hospital where I worked, so I hadn't actually set foot on that turf often.

It felt truly weird to enter the hospital as a patient, carrying my MRI, being greeted by former colleagues. There were a lot of gray hairs now, but we were still the same people in many ways, and familiar expressions and idiosyncrasies aroused the past sufficiently to make me feel that my case was really someone else's. I had spoken with the adult radiation oncologist many times over the years, so we were quite informal with one another. He bypassed the resident's preliminary exam and skipped the rectal. We discussed my case, a rehash of old stuff, plus the case-experience specific to that institution, new stuff. It was his impression that the statistics for surgery and radiation were comparable. He was not a big fan of seeds, but told me that his implanters were using a high dose temporary implant technique. I had read a bit about that, but it was clear that data were preliminary and no one could say whether it was any better than permanent seeds or radiation alone. He implied that I should have whole pelvis radiation, but without strong conviction, and he suggested that radiation could be delivered at any of three possible regional locations, including my local hospital across the street from my office. I was happy to see the old crowd, but I left harboring more confusion than before. And this was before Boston.

The East Coast connection was derived strangely and took on even more bizarre twists as it evolved. A local friend of mine called to say that a former student of his, a nonphysician, was working at a well-known radiation unit in Boston. Would I like to speak with him? I said yes, of course, and was even more interested when I heard the name of the physician in charge. He was well regarded, especially as an expert in prostate cancer radiation; I had seen his name on numerous papers. His name also seemed vaguely familiar, a name from the past. He had been at the same medical center where I did a five-month externship in surgery, some thirty years before.

With some hesitation, I wrote to him questioning whether our paths had indeed crossed and detailing my current situation. Boston has an aura of formality lacking in the West. I never thought I would get to speak with this expert directly, but when I called some days later, he got on the phone and we chatted. We figured out our connection. I had written my first medical paper during that externship, a case report about a rare surgical disorder. This very same man, then a surgery resident and now a very well-known, respected radiation oncologist, had treated the patient I described in that paper. The coincidence seemed uncanny to me. It felt as though I was being guided in some strange way. Turning to my problem, he laid out his opinion. Radiation, when given at a proper dose and in a proper fashion was every bit as good, if not better than surgery. Seed implantation was perhaps a passing fad, or at least, an unproven technique. Various radiation beams related to X rays, such as proton or neutron beams, might possibly reduce side effects and allow for even higher doses to the tumor, but the research was still in progress. Of course, there could be no long-term outcome data for many years. The work was being conducted at his institution and in Southern California. I could come to Boston, if I wished. He couldn't tell me whether it was worth doing, but he would be glad to treat me if I did.

When I queried him about choosing between the radiation oncologist at my local hospital across the street and the university medical center radiation oncologist, he said (paraphrasing), "You have one of the ten leading prostate radiation oncologists in the country fifteen miles away and you would consider having your treatment elsewhere?" How could I not follow his recommendations to the letter? Well, eventually I did and I didn't. For the time being, I continued my research.

A friend who did not have prostate cancer, but had been struggling with other prostate problems for years, told me about a colleague of his, a research psychologist, who had been recently diagnosed with prostate cancer. This man had done exhaustive investigation on his own and was currently receiving radiation and seeds. I gave him a call and we met for lunch. He was quite intense. One could feel his thoroughness. He had pored over papers, was well-versed in statistics, and told me that most of the published studies had major flaws. He saw the pitfalls involved in trying to compare modalities when outcome was a matter of many years and changes in therapies were sometimes a matter of months. His prostate cancer numbers were better than mine, yet he had rejected surgery. His overriding concern had been the risk of suffering needless loss of sexual function and continence. We talked about his choice of venue for external beam and seed implants. He had made his decisions based on a combination of convenience and experience. He did not want to drive thirty miles a day for the external beam, but he would fly to Seattle for the implants. It was encouraging to follow his progress through treatment phases, because he suffered virtually no ill effects from his treatments. I began to feel a sense of occasional optimism. Perhaps it wouldn't be too bad after all.

Along the way, these consultations and meetings were peppered with evening stints on the Internet and calls to physicians and acquaintances who had also had prostate cancer. One man, a colleague in internal medicine at the hospital where I see my newborn patients, had had surgery at the university medical center. He reported that he was well and felt himself cured. But when he described his actual experience, it turned out that he had had a series of complications that made my knees shake. Another colleague, a therapist, met me in his study. I had seen

him in a hospital bed five years before recovering from his prostatectomy. He had told me then that it wasn't too bad, and here
he was, disease free years later. I remembered thinking five years
earlier, "That could be me in five years."

I spoke with the wife of another prostate cancer patient who
had had surgery fraught with complications and a protracted
recovery. I also spoke with a physician who had had bad luck
with seeds implanted by experts in Seattle and who had to
catheterize himself for nighttime urinary obstruction over an
eight-month period. Another friend who had had radiation alone,
finally felt well after three years of low-level diarrhea and dietary
intolerances. A prominent and dedicated local pediatric colleague
graciously invited me to his home to chat and told me he chose
seeds because it involved the least amount of time lost from work!
He missed all of five days, I believe, including a weekend. No
one who saw him at weekly Grand Rounds would ever have sus-
pected anything had ever been wrong.

Another phone call to the friend of a friend gave me a picture of treatment with hormones and radiation. We talked a bit
about loss of sexual urge and other potential complications. As I
continued to read the complication rate tables in the research
papers I collected, I realized that there was simply no predicting
the future in this business. It was clear that no form of treatment
for prostate cancer offered a free lunch. For any given complication, I might as well toss a coin to figure out my own likelihood
of encountering it. A published statistical likelihood of 10 percent
could seem large or a small depending on my mood of the hour.

Weeks had passed since the biopsy, weeks marked by much
agonizing and indecision. I felt comfortable with all of the local

radiation experts I had consulted. Emails were being written and answered, filtering through my conscious and unconscious thought processes like a witch's brew. Not wishing to further delay treatment and slip into watchful waiting, I had begun hormone injections. The consensus seemed to be that two or three months of treatment before radiation and an undetermined amount of time during and after treatment might be of benefit. Depriving the prostate of testosterone would cause some cell death and shrink the size of the gland. The plan was strongly advocated by some, grudgingly acknowledged as possibly effective by others. I also had a consultation with the university-based urology oncologists. I thought they might offer a fairly unbiased evaluation of my chances and the treatment options. Urology oncologists usually have to wrestle with treatment failures, patients who have relapsed after surgery or radiation. Some scoffed at my decision to see these physicians at such an early stage. Yet it proved invaluable. We went over the Partin tables, which take stage and Gleason score and generate likelihood of cancer spread. I had a greater than 60 percent chance that the tumor had penetrated the capsule of the prostate gland. The oncologist recommended hormones, radiation, and possibly seeds.

Things were beginning to gel in my mind. Then I got sidetracked once again. I ran into a pediatric colleague of mine, a very bright guy, something of a nonconformist with his own ideas about medicine. He had experience in biostatistics and clinical pediatric cancer trials before becoming a general pediatrician. We chatted about matters, both pediatric and personal. When my partner was having her gynecological problems, he had mentioned some findings about the hormonal milieu surrounding menopause and what he saw as a dangerous emphasis on isolated estrogen replacement. At the time, we had been talking about breast cancer, and he had mentioned the name of another medical voice in the wilderness, a lone ranger proponent of so-called natural progesterones. Now that the issue was my prostate cancer, he again mentioned the name of this physician whom he held in high esteem and suggested I give the man a call, to discuss this hormone in the context of prostate cancer. I did just that. I had a lovely and informative discussion with an individual who basically did not have to give me the time of day. He was now pretty much retired, although he continued to be active, giving talks all over the country about his theories and findings. The only information he could offer me on prostate cancer was anecdotal, including a series of positive success stories, mostly involving men who responded to natural—that is nonsynthesized—progesterone after their physicians declared them incurable. Ordinarily, I would immediately dismiss this kind of information in my mind, but this man's grounding in endocrinology and his physiological arguments seemed sound and impressive.

He told me that a clinical trial was about to begin in southern California, based on preliminary test-tube results suggesting that progesterone could be quite active against prostate cancer. I left our conversation with two names, two more contacts, and I followed up on them. The first was a doctor with metastatic prostate cancer who had been taking progesterone and had a dramatic prolonged clinical response plus a drop in his PSA. He was thrilled, but I knew I couldn't do much with the information. His story was encouraging to hear, but I couldn't very well hang my hat on his individual short-term experience. The second contact was a research scientist who was about to launch the clinical trials investigating nonsynthesized progesterone. This conversation was also encouraging, but clearly, it would be some time before there would be any data.

This lead was typical of other nonconventional ones. The result was an exposure to tantalizing, intriguing, but untested information, leading to novel approaches that were appealing mostly because they were less invasive than standard therapy, but also in their promise of the possibility of better results in cases such as mine. I was sufficiently impressed and diverted to buy a tube of progesterone cream. It continues to sit, unopened, on a shelf in my medicine cabinet. Every now and then, I still look at that tube, check its expiration date, and wonder how things are progressing in southern California.

In fact, I had also encountered the outlying opinion of one Los Angeles oncologist who thought that prostate cancer could be controlled comparably by testosterone deprivation alone, that is, without surgery or radiation. No other mainstream physician involved in the treatment of prostate cancer agreed with this maverick and, unfortunately, he had not published peer-reviewed data to corroborate his opinion. Yet his arguments, hotly presented at medical meetings and displayed verbatim on his Web page, were very intriguing. He was not available for phone or email discussions. I considered a 400-mile trip south for yet another consultation, but decided against it. During my training, I had known an oncologist who delivered his prognoses and pronouncements based on personal experience rather than on published data. Force of personality, charm, and optimism led many to follow his advice, and rarely did those patients fare better than those who had by-the-book therapy. I didn't want to place myself in this vulnerable position, and I knew that even if this person was persuasive and showed me his data, the lack of peer review would render it suspect.

Nevertheless, in my compulsive fashion, mostly to corroborate my impression about hormone-alone therapy, I called yet another prostate specialist in southern California, an oncologist who ran a prostate cancer Web page on the Internet. We had trained at the same institution and knew the same people. Following the professional preliminaries, a short, crisp general discussion about prostate cancer ensued. Some time later, I called him again to check out a small point and he curtly informed me that he did not offer professional courtesy, so I would have to come see him if I wanted to continue the discussion, or why not just talk to the experts in my area? I had hardly taken advantage of this person and had become accustomed to, and reliant on, the understanding of professional colleagues. This one negative experience smarted and made me angry. It seemed so mercenary and humiliating.

Under pressure to make decisions, I began to formulate a date to begin radiation, still not having decided between external beam alone, pelvic versus conformal radiation, radiation plus seeds, or who would do what and where would I have it done? Timely serendipity surfaced once again. The annual American Academy of Pediatrics meetings were being held locally, and I decided to attend for one day, partly to maintain my educational credits and partly to see an old friend and colleague. We met at the end of the day and I told her of my situation. This friend, long a heroine of mine, suggested I call a urologist colleague of hers to get another opinion because "they do things a little differently in

Canada." I looked him up on the Internet, read some abstracts, and found that they did indeed do things differently. His group had been prescribing long periods of testosterone deprivation hormone therapy before surgery. The aim was to provide maximum apoptosis early on—this being tumor death by a kind of hormonal starvation. I was especially intrigued because my research had already led me to this phenomenon of apoptosis, and it tied in with some principles of treatment of malignancies in general.

I called the urologist in Canada after reading his published papers. It is amazing how dropping the right name leads to access. It took a few calls, but I soon had my personal phone consultation. What I learned was that this urologist had used an approach I had already been contemplating after absorbing all the literature I had collected over the previous weeks. Prostate cancer cells depend on testosterone. Why not use that fact to reduce the number of viable tumor cells as much as possible before initiating radiation or surgery? Why not use this process akin to starvation, this apoptosis, to early advantage? The argument that prostate cancer cells eventually become resistant to hormone deprivation or that one should "save" hormone deprivation for cases of relapse did not impress me. I recalled my years treating children with leukemia. The single factor that best correlated with success was a small initial amount of tumor, or the ability to reduce the tumor dramatically to undetectable levels at the onset of treatment. Fostering apoptosis sounded like the way to go.

The group in Canada used testosterone blockade for about eight months before doing a radical prostatectomy. Applying a variety of special stains at the time of the biopsy and on the tissue obtained at surgery, they were able to compare the before and after state of the tumor. They found marked reductions in tumor size that exceeded what one might expect with shorter hormone treatments. In fact, the lower the PSA was driven, the less identifiable tumor was left behind. Of course, no one could be absolutely sure that the process of apoptosis was complete. The cancer regression might have left some minute nests of viable tumor cells in the anatomical areas they had once occupied. But the marked regression of tumor at surgery was encouraging, and there seemed to be a direct correlation between disease-free survival and the lowest PSA attained during hormonal testosterone blockade. When I asked about the same approach in patients who selected radiation therapy, this urologist burst my bubble yet again by bluntly stating that he had never seen a patient cured of prostate cancer by radiation, so none of his patients went that route. That forceful pronouncement was hard to swallow. So I might follow his guidelines in one aspect, but not in another. I just didn't want to undergo that surgery.

The search was now on for a radiation oncologist who had incorporated prolonged testosterone deprivation up front. One potential physician in Quebec served as a reminder that not everyone wishes to be contacted. I must have placed half a dozen phone calls to him, to his assistants, and to his secretary. I even tried out some of my rusty French, all to no avail. A pathologist in Vancouver was kind and helpful, but he had no experience beyond that summarized by the urologist in his group. I finally reached a radiation oncologist in the Canadian midwest who had patients on long-term testosterone deprivation followed by radiation. She was encouraging and thought the approach reasonable, but she had no long-term or published outcome data.

I had finally arrived at a decision based on all these consultations and some others I have not summarized, and I told my close family members what I intended to do. Some were afraid that I would never have the radiation, that I would use the prolonged hormone treatment interval for further procrastination. I was amazed that I had chosen relatively uncharted ground. Yet I knew that I would follow the hormone treatment to an appropriate end, and then proceed to the next step. I was not relieved or overly confident, but I set out on this chosen path.

In retrospect, I had actually followed the path first casually suggested by my own urologist: "Just decide between surgery and radiation." But my decision had been long in coming, based on my own convoluted and compulsive manner. Was I wrong to go to such lengths, to drag those near me through such protracted vacillation and uncertainty? It will be years before I know the long-term success of my treatment. But I felt better for having done an extensive investigation, and for making a decision, though it differed from suggestions proposed by most of my consulting physicians. Curiously, as some validation of my conclusions, the path I chose to follow has subsequently been adopted by a number of experts in the field. For better or for worse, I had put together a choice for my treatment. Now and forever more, I would have to live with my decision.

Chapter Six

The Balance Unbalanced

Once I decided to have radiation rather than a radical prostatectomy, it was fairly easy to move toward treatment with hormones, specifically with anti-androgens. Remember that most prostate cancer cells need testosterone. Without the presence of this hormone, the programmed death of cancer cells is accelerated. Testosterone belongs to the group of male sex hormones called androgens. While these androgens are associated with desirable, as well as undesirable, male sex characteristics such as facial hair and aggression, they are not unique to men. Testosterone is also present in women, albeit in far smaller quantities. Throughout my treatment, I was ever reminded of the overlap between male and female by the power and peculiarities of the so-called sex hormones. Above all, hormones normally acquire their own state of balance in our bodies, one resembling choreographed equilibrium.

These hormones have an important role in the evolution and treatment of prostate cancer. It is possible both to reduce the amount of circulating androgens, mostly testosterone, and to interfere with the steps that render testosterone useful to targeted tissues. Think of a lock and a key. To prevent a lock from opening, you can either take away the key or change its configuration so it no longer fits the lock. Or, in theory, you can alter the lock so it no longer accepts the key. All of these approaches apply to the development of drugs that disrupt the process by which testosterone encourages the growth of prostate cancer cells.

Prostate cancer is only one of a number of tumors that are characterized as being hormone dependent. Another prominent example is breast cancer. Curiously, there is substantial overlap between these two cancers, both in their increase over the past years and in the manner in which they behave. Much of this similarity has yet to be explored or explained. It has been said that prostate cancer now is to men what breast cancer was to women fifteen years ago. It is on the rise as a diagnosis that men think about, feel threatened by, and are acutely aware of. Its treatment is still relatively primitive because so little is known about how it behaves and what is likely to reverse it. The association of both breast and prostate with sexual identity is obvious, and the tissues are embryologically related and share some characteristics. We are in the infancy of understanding the interaction of genes, hormones, the environment, and certain malignancies. Some day in the future, therapy strategies may take advantage of the hormonal similarities of certain malignancies, which may also provide clues about their origins.

Despite our relative ignorance about cancers, the impact of androgen deprivation on prostate cancer has been known for years. As is the case with many approaches, we determine its effectiveness from studies carried out in advanced cases, those in which the cancer has spread. One of the effective treatments for advanced metastasic prostate cancer has been the administration of estrogen. Estrogen is a female counterpart of testosterone. It defines many female sex characteristics, but is also present in men in smaller quantities. Another long-standing treatment option for advanced cases of prostate cancer has been castration, removal of the testosterone-producing testicles. The drama and finality of this step can be hard hitting. Years ago, removal of the ovaries was a comparable method of treating advanced breast cancer. In some ways, the parallels are striking.

Dramatic remissions, identified by decreased pain and a reduced extent of metastases, frequently follow the initiation of androgen deprivation therapy. Unfortunately, the disease invariably returns sooner or later, and the hormonal manipulations typically cease to work. Until very recently, it was thought that the cancer cells simply learned to do without testosterone. The current thinking is that the genetic changes or mutations that render a cell insensitive to the effect of hormones are rare events; they are more likely to occur on a random basis in the presence of extensive cancer. In other words, if such a mutation occurs randomly once in every ten thousand cell divisions in cells throughout the body, a testosterone-resistance mutation is more likely to occur if there are a million cancer cells present as opposed to a hundred, simply because more cells are dividing at any given moment.

During my research effort, I came across studies that showed an advantage for men with advanced cancer who received anti-androgen hormone treatment over longer periods of time following conventional radiation treatment of the primary tumor. I also saw data that suggested this kind of hormone treatment could successfully be given intermittently, six months on and six months off. The person who would do my external beam radiation therapy—yet another world famous physician whose viewpoint was not to be discounted—believed that hormones should only be given over long periods of time to those who carried a high risk of relapse following standard radiation. He was dubious about intermittent hormone treatment and presented the analogy of antibiotics to justify his position. It has long been held that resistance is encouraged by suboptimal doses and intermittent administration. Yet I knew from my pediatric literature that this doctrine was changing. Shorter antibiotic courses seem to have no negative impact on drug resistance. A wide variety of doses and means of administration do not seem to have an impact. What matters with antibiotics is how extensively they are used in a community, because bacteria have evolved to a range of sensitivities in the antibiotic era, and resistance depends on the passage from one child to another of the relatively more resistant strains. So it seemed to me that the analogy might not apply. And in my experience with pediatric oncology patients, resistance to chemotherapy agents seemed to depend more on something that happened to the cancer than on the way in which the chemotherapeutic agent was given. Of course, I was also aware that hormones are neither antibiotic agents nor chemotherapy. A simple analogy might not be convincing.

It occurred to me that a better analogy might have been that of leukemia, with which I was quite familiar. When leukemia first becomes apparent, the number of malignant cells, referred to as the tumor burden, is very high. The first phase of treatment, called induction, aims to destroy as many cells as possible. Over the years, increasingly vigorous agents have been used to try to achieve this goal. If induction has been achieved, standard techniques no longer detect leukemia cells in the body, and this state is called remission. It is not called a cure, because we know that some cancer cells persist in the body, and these cancer cells often reside in locations they favor, termed sanctuaries. There follows another phase of treatment called consolidation, during which treatment is directed at cells hiding in sanctuaries. If remission continues, maintenance therapy is given for a number of years, during which it is assumed that the chemotherapy, combined with the body's own defense mechanisms can eradicate remaining tumor cells. But did it make sense to apply principles derived from the treatment of leukemia to prostate cancer?

I also knew that the evolution of cancer treatment often progresses from lower to higher doses and from less aggressive to more aggressive approaches. Until a satisfactory balance is achieved between destroying the tumor and destroying the patient, cure rates tend to be on the low side. More aggressive treatment is chosen only after it has been demonstrated that a milder therapy plan has failed.

Although leukemia and prostate cancer certainly differ, some characteristics are shared by most malignancies. What seemed to make sense to me from the leukemia analogy is that maximum destruction of cancer cells should be sought at the onset. Hormone-induced apoptosis appeared to be the best way of achieving this goal for prostate cancer once it was determined that surgery was not likely to remove all of the tumor. By contrast, the approach typically taken in solid tumor oncology (cancer of the lung, for example), namely surgical "de-bulking" followed by mop-up radiation, seemed undesirable to me for two reasons. First, most solid tumors do not provide a hormone-responsive option. Second, effective chemotherapy regimens, the mainstay of this kind of treatment for tumors like breast cancer, have not yet proved to be very effective for prostate cancer.

This reasoning combined with a nagging opinion from that lone vocal maverick prostate oncologist lauding the merits of hormone therapy alone and the encouraging studies from Vancouver led me to favor a longer initial period of anti-androgen treatment for myself. This decision, once again, led to even more choices. What seemed most effective, according to at least some published studies, was a combination of anti-androgen approaches termed complete androgen blockade. Throughout this whole analytic process, I kept wondering what I would be like, what would happen to me, in the course of this pharmacological assault on my masculinity. On bad days, I feared I would regress to the very first stages of adolescence, those years in which the girls become taller than the boys and more physically developed. On good days, I was able to put the matter into balanced perspective remembering this treatment phase would be time limited and perhaps the most innocuous of my treatment modalities.

At this point, I need to pause in the telling of my story to explain hormone therapy further. It is important to have at least a rudimentary idea about how these hormones work. Many hormonal systems function by using a finely tuned mechanism called a *feedback loop*. When the hypothalamus in the brain senses a need for a specific hormone, it stimulates the pituitary gland to

produce a first set of hormones; these stimulate the gland responsible for producing the needed secondary hormone. Thus the brain
can stimulate the thyroid gland to produce thyroid hormone, the
pancreas to produce insulin, the adrenal gland to produce corti-
costeroid hormones, the testicle to produce testosterone, and so
forth. The target organ may produce and release one or a number of related hormones, which may act on other organs or may
be metabolized to yet other hormones with differing activities.
The circulating hormones register their presence in the pituitary
gland, which, amazingly enough, can turn its selective spigots on
or off as required, depending on whether there is too much or
too little of a particular circulating hormone.

Medications have been developed to interrupt this system and
trick a man's body into blocking the effects of testosterone. One
group of medications stimulates the pituitary gland so it exhausts
its supply of the hormone that signals the need for testosterone
production. These medications are called LHRH agonists/antag-
onists. LHRH stands for luteinizing hormone releasing hormone,
and its name actually derives from its effect on the female ovary.
The hormonal crossover between the sexes becomes apparent once
again. The same hormone that causes an ovary to release a sub-
stance that governs a woman's menstrual cycle also functions to
release testosterone in a man. If the testicle and the adrenal gland
do not receive a hormonal signal from the brain's pituitary gland,
they will not produce the body's testosterone. The most common
LHRH agonists are leuprolide (Lupron) and goserelin (Zoladex).
These are given by injection—a long needle, deep into the but-
tock or thigh muscle. The shot is typically given once a month,
although longer lasting depot versions are also available. The

trade-off here is between the frequency of the injections and the reliability of circulating high levels of the LHRH agonist.

Because LHRH agonists first stimulate then deplete testosterone, men may experience a flare reaction when they first begin receiving injections. This flare can cause difficulty urinating or increased bone pain in patients who have bone metastases. Subsequently, as testosterone decreases, men are apt to have hot flashes and breast soreness. Loss of sex drive is both a curious and powerful consequence of androgen depletion, but it tends to occur gradually with repeated injections. One thinks perhaps it won't happen, but it does, and it is quite a shock when it does. Thanks a lot, I thought to myself. When I began experiencing these inevitable side effects, they became a bit of a joke between me and my officemate. She was in the throes of menopause, having serious hot flashes, and had recently had her own sexuality threatened by breast cancer. We sweated and mopped brows together and exchanged knowing giggles, but I must say that she had a harder time with this than I did. Compared to her hot flashes, mine were distinctly on the mild side.

Another group of commonly used hormone antagonists are the anti-androgens. Common anti-androgen agents are flutamide (Eulexin), bicalutamide (Casodex), and nilutamide (Nilandron). In the lock and key analogy, these medications work by tampering with the lock. On the surface of the target cell—the cell to be influenced by the hormone—is a receptor, (the lock). The anti-androgens block the cell's receptor for testosterone. Each of these medications has its own set of characteristics, advantages, and disadvantages. The longest clincial experience is with flutamide, but it must be taken, hence remembered, three times a day. Bicalutamide can cause heart problems. Nilutamide is less readily available and is incompatible with alcohol. All can cause varying degrees of diarrhea (20 percent of patients) and abnormal liver function (10 percent of patients). Once again, there is no free lunch in this business!

Another approach is to block the metabolism of testosterone, in which an enzyme converts it to dihydroxytestosterone, a more active androgen. One of the drugs that blocks this enzyme, finistride (Proscar) is used to treat enlargement of the prostate gland. One would think it should be active against prostate cancer, but this has not yet been shown to be the case. This is one of the nicer drugs for an older guy, because finistride is also used to slow down the process of balding.

When combinations of these hormones and medications are used, the effect is called maximal or complete androgen blockade. In this case, there is a rational way to begin. First, an anti-androgen is prescribed to block the flare effect of the LHRH agonist. A couple of weeks later, the first injection of the LHRH agonist is given. Some throw in the finistride as well, because one of the aims is to shrink the size of the prostate to make it a better target for the X-ray beam. It was time to choose my LHRH agonist and anti-androgen and proceed. My doctors had no preference. Had I been just anyone, I might have been handed a prescription, told to take the medication, and return for injections. But I already identified myself as a medical auto-micromanager. So I was asked what I would like to do rather than told. My choices were Lupron once a month, or as a depot injection once every three months, or Zoladex in its stead, and the three times a day Eulexin, or the once a day Casodex, and yes or no on the Proscar.

Nilandron was not available at the time. You can figure out for yourself how many different combinations were possible. So here is how I decided. I went with Lupron once a month, first, because it was more readily available and used more commonly, and monthly, because this spacing might provide more even dosing than a larger amount left to seep into my body over a longer period of time. I went with Casodex, because I thought I would forget to take medication three times a day. And I went with Proscar, because why not?

I started to take my medicine, had my first blood test two weeks later, and then reported for my first injection. Because this stuff is so expensive, the nurses could not order it from the pharmacy until I showed my face. Each Lupron injection costs the pharmacy about $500. This amount, the average wholesale price (AWP), can be revealed by any pharmacist. One has to wonder what happens to the poor gentleman who is uninsured and can't afford such medication. I found out the answer to this riddle with my first EOB. The letters EOB stand for "explanation of benefits," and a privately insured patient receives this information from his insurer telling him what was charged, what the insurance company paid, and what residual the patient owes. With the advent of HMO medicine, most patients no longer receive an EOB, because everything is prepaid at a cut rate. Hence, compensatory price increases are written into the billing process to try to recover the short fall. Each injection I received was charged at more than $1,300! The insurance company paid half, and I was charged an additional $180 per injection. The remainder was to be written off by the hospital. The relatively minor $180 out-of-pocket expense adds up quickly when it is billed once a month. The tax benefits are zero if you have a relatively high income. And why should a person with cancer have to think about any of this anyway? But that is a political discussion.

I had applied a prescription EMLA anesthetic patch two hours before the injection to numb the site. I don't care for pain, and I always avoid shots like the plague. In fact, when I was young, I had a very low opinion of my own pediatrician who gave his own shots. The oncology nurses were fabulous. Nursing can be a fairly thankless job, taking orders from physicians who may or may not be pleasant or appreciative, doing procedures that hurt, and getting very little credit for treatment successes. Yet all the nurses I encountered in the oncology outpatient clinic were cheerful, pleasant, and encouraging. None smirked at my EMLA. They warned me before the poke and asked me afterward how it was. It never hurt much with the EMLA patch applied, and I never forgot the EMLA, so I don't know how it would have been without it. Every time I got one of these shots, I thought of the way Tom Hanks pronounced the anatomical word, butt-tock in the movie Forrest Gump. That provided me a puny inner smile on an otherwise unpleasant occasion.

My doctor called me a few days after the first Lupron injection. My liver function tests were slightly elevated. "Let's repeat them in two weeks," he said. On repeat, they were somewhat higher. This meant I might be in the 8 to 10 percent of men who develop liver abnormalities from anti-androgens. Why me? I was upset because I had read that complete hormonal blockade was more effective than partial blockade. I immediately felt I was destined to fall into a bad luck category, already having discovered unexpectedly extensive cancer and now developing a relatively rare complication right at the onset of my treatment. I complained to my officemate, and she suggested that I consult her herbal- ist/acupuncturist, someone well regarded in the medical commu- nity. In fact, he was involved in joint research with breast cancer oncologists at the university medical center—a mainstream acupuncturist!

My officemate had taken, and was still taking, an herbal sub- stance. She had become a queen of broccoli sprouts and soy milk. She had joined a support group. She was practicing stress reduc- tion. So here we were, two scientifically trained physicians thrust into the world of alternative or complementary medicine because of the limitations of our own discipline. Where would I fit into all this, the Great Skeptic and Rationalist? I gave her acupunc- turist a call and we talked.

What I encountered was a soft-spoken, thoughtful, and well- informed individual. He followed my reasoning, listened to my misgivings, gently reminded me not to ignore conventional ther- apy, and talked about herbs and acupuncture with an endearing and refreshing combination of assurance and humility. While the effects of many herbs seemed documented to his satisfaction, much remained unknown. Our conversations happened to coincide with the publication of a paper evaluating an alternative prostate can- cer treatment, PC-SPES, in *The New England Journal of Medicine*. This article had documented both the effectiveness and hazards of herbal substances, revealing the emergence of an incompletely studied yet potentially helpful drug that had not passed through the customary maze and hurdles of the pharmaceutical regulato- ry process. We talked about radiation, vitamins, herbs, and acupuncture and decided to meet. Over lunch at a local Thai restaurant, he suggested an herbal mixture as a possible treatment for the liver toxicity Casodex was causing me. I had also mentioned tension headaches obviously related to the distress over the liver toxicity and the decision-making process in which I was currently over-engaged. He said acupuncture might help. What the hell, I thought, as I called his receptionist and made a formal appointment.

When I arrived, I realized I was in for a novel experience. The setup was superficially not unlike a medical one, but everything had a different cast. There was a reception area, including a desk with a computer terminal, behind which sat an informally dressed woman. But all of this was surrounded by couches and Eastern, that is Asian, accoutrements, health magazines, acupuncture point charts, Buddha statuettes, and such.

After what seemed like a long wait in the company of a couple of women whose head scarves and knitted caps revealed the nature of their illness, my new friend emerged and we went into a back room. It looked like a standard examination room, but missing were the scales, blood pressure cuffs, and medical instruments. Treatment materials seemed to consist only of a flat mat on an exam table and some alcohol and cotton balls. He carefully reviewed a lengthy history I had been asked to fill out while waiting. This encompassed much more than the usual symptom and family history questions. He asked about the usual problems concerning headaches, vision, hearing, stomach, urine, or limbs. But there were also questions about lifestyle, sensitivities, work and sleep patterns, matters that are often considered "nonmedical" in import. Of course, everything is potentially medical if you take the time to make appropriate connections.

I was becoming holistic despite myself. We briefly touched on the traditional Chinese approach to symptoms and body functions. This was definitely a foreign language to me, and I maintained respectful emotional distance, while I tried to mount participatory enthusiasm. The recurring bug-a-boos were ones I had encountered some years prior when I had engaged in a lively disagreement with a group of homeopaths who decried routine immunization. The traditional Chinese medicine approach incorporated well-defined principles, but was also highly individualized, depending on the patient's response. If something didn't seem to work, it was modified in accordance with principles and experience. If something did work, the practitioner could not tell you precisely why nor could he reproduce the same effect reliably using the same exact means in another patient with the same diagnosis.

Some alternative or holistic approaches could angle towards another slippery slope to which I had been exposed during my tenure as a pediatric oncologist. There had been forms of individualized "treatment" that were said to depend on a patient's positive attitude for their efficacy. Visualization techniques, for example, might not be effective if the participant did not believe they would work. Failure could thus always be attributed to a deficiency or lack on the part of the patient as opposed to the "treatment!" This brought such alternative techniques dangerously close to faith healing. This is not to decry faith. There is data suggesting that faith helps the healing process. But faith alone cannot be held responsible for a patient's health. What was proposed for me did not seem to carry this caveat, so I permitted my innate resistance to give way to personal experimentation. I was about to enter an anecdotal world, one devoid of much truth in the standard medical model.

My acupuncturist/herbalist and I chatted amiably and comfortably. It was amazing how unthreatening this encounter felt. I had the sense of healing as opposed to treatment because the process seemed so mild and personal. Instead of pigeon-holing the individual's problems and symptoms into a set system of diagnoses, algorithms, and treatment protocols, the practitioner listens carefully to the composite story, elicits a wide range of characteristics that define the patient's overall health, and builds a picture of the individual seated before him, taking into account every aspect of that person's life. The physical examination makes no sense if approached using traditional medical criteria. My skin color was observed. My pulse was taken, not to count a number per minute, but rather to assess qualities of that pulse that I could not imagine evaluating objectively. My tongue was studied. Because I have what is called a geographic tongue, one naturally endowed with furrows and irregularities, I wondered what was being gleaned from this exercise. My practitioner then pronounced me to have indicators of anti-androgen effect, which of course he knew in advance. Yet when I queried him further, the indicators he mentioned appeared to have some plausibility. During all of this, I continued to have a sense of calm, of a positive effort directed completely toward me as an individual living being, the sole recipient of this attention. This was not a guru effect.

My practitioner was born Israeli. He was kind, but did not exude mysterious charisma. There were no piercing glances, soft lights, New Age sounds, white silk clothes, or sandals. As I expected, he now suggested I try acupuncture for the tension headaches.

While I do not have needle aversion, I don't do well with pain, and it took a bit of mental steeling to recall that these ultra-thin needles are said not to be painful. I lay down on the couch, prepared to take my medicine.

With obvious expertise, my practitioner cleaned the designated areas and twirled solid needles into the webs between my thumb and forefingers and between the great toe and its neighbor on both my feet. I felt a sensation of tingling and warmth, exactly as described by friends of mine who had had acupuncture. I felt relaxed. Then came the catch. I was to lie still for twenty minutes! The needles might be painful if I moved, so be careful and just relax. I do not belong to those for whom twenty minutes of inactivity comes naturally. As the door closed, my nose began to itch as my psyche objected to immobility. But lie still I did, maintaining my composure by playing long movements of symphonic music in my head. At times like this, music becomes my narcotic, my avenue to disassociation. Toward the end, I actually felt pretty good, although I was anxious to have the needles out and be able to scratch my nose.

The acupuncture session concluded, we next turned our attention to my liver toxicity. An herbal mixture was suggested. The computer generated a "prescription" in response to Chinese terms dictated to the receptionist. This prescription, containing numerous ingredients, emerged from the printer as a lengthy printout resembling a complicated dinner recipe. The big difference, I was told, was that this recipe would taste vile. I was to have four teaspoons mixed in warm water after breakfast, lunch, and dinner, potentially ruining any lingering pleasure from these meals. When I asked about toxicity, I was assured that these ingredients were

all common, well-tolerated herbs without the potential for adul-
teration by unwanted substances, such as arsenic. These herbal
ingredients were known to promote liver health and beneficial
stimulation of the immune system.

Now, the term "system" rankles me. While digestive system
and immune system are terms that have identifiable meaning for
physicians, the layman often uses the word "system" in a very
nebulous fashion. It appears in parlance as though the human
body were a composite of various mechanical systems joined
together in balanced health as an anatomic and physiological jig-
saw puzzle, having the unfortunate potential for missing or mis-
matched pieces.

Patients ask me whether frequent colds are a sign of a "weak
immune system," and what can they give a child to strengthen
"her immune system"? Even worse, parents ask whether an event,
illness, medication, or voyage, will stress "his system"? What system might that be? Any physiological function does not stand in
isolation, but is comprised of numerous interacting elements, many
of which are specifically identified. The term "system" reawak-
ens an old saw promulgated by those skeptical of traditional medicine, by invoking and criticizing reductionism, that is, the
emphasis on small elements as opposed to the whole being, or
holism. Yet smaller elements are easier to study and therefore better and more reliably understood. The big picture is valid, but
slippery and hard to define. Stress is bad for you, but it affects
everyone differently. One is not much the wiser to learn that stress
is bad for "the system." So when an herb is touted as benefiting
the immune "system," I am left wondering what part of the immune
system that might be. I had to consciously permit curiosity and a

new cavalier attitude to overcome years of medical training so I could try out this herbal stuff.

It was the inability of known medical practice to influence the liver toxicity of the Casodex that led me to try the herbs. I wanted complete hormonal blockade if I could get it, and was frightened about the prospect of losing a component of the anti-androgens if my liver function worsened. I was less worried about toxicity of the herbs than I should have been. Recent data has suggested that many of these preparations are hardly harmless. It seems the country of origin relates mightily to the purity and uniformity of the product. Here we have Eastern medicines that are produced with better quality control by Western European manufacturers!

I live in an area where herbal and homeopathic remedies are readily available in venues ranging from authentic Chinese establishments to New Age shops to designated aisles in yuppie supermarkets. But I was sent to a particular dispensary run by a Swiss man who obtains quality herbs directly from China and safely compounds the mixtures himself. So now the care and precision of the West was to be combined with the authenticity of the East. I had come to realize that in order to conduct this adventure, I had to dismiss any doubts or sinister thoughts about kickbacks, and place myself completely in the hands of my herbalist. I hadn't a clue as to what was going on here, so I might as well cultivate some trust and hope for the best. This was akin to an airplane flight. I simply couldn't pilot the trip. I had to sit back and relax.

I handed over my prescription, that incomprehensible list of Chinese words. Within the shop, shelves were lined with various concoctions and small bags of root-like substances were scattered throughout. The place smelled musty, as though I was in a forest. On the bulletin board were business cards advertising any form of therapy one might care to imagine—massage, reflexology, music therapy, magnets, you name it. Classical music wafted through the establishment. The proprietor was pleasant and attacked the prescription with his assistant. Preparation involved shouting out and measuring each ingredient, adding it to the gemisch in a blender, and giving it a whirr. The resulting powder was funneled into three plastic bottles that were labeled with directions. The process was not reassuring since the mixture was concocted rapidly and seemingly without great care to exact measurements. It appeared thrown together, but I had been forewarned by my officemate who had gone through the same process, so I retained my equanimity throughout. Fifteen minutes later, I emerged from this quintessentially nonmedical experience with three containers of what looked like dirt, but cost close to $50, credit card happily accepted, thank you.

If ever there was a good example of "the medicine has to taste bad in order for it to work," this herbal mixture was it. I would drop three of the four prescribed teaspoons full into a glass of warm water and stir as though my life depended on it. The brew smelled bad and tasted worse. I needed a water or juice chaser afterward and was never able to manage the prescribed four teaspoons that would have constituted a proper dose. This was partly due to its vileness and partly to loose stools, a known consequence of these herbs. As the days continued, I often missed a dose here or there. I am sure this lapse of memory was psychological in origin. I stuck it out, though, for a fair trial, and anticipated my next blood test with a measure of sly curiosity. My prescribing physician did not know about this undertaking.

The long and short of it is that following acupuncture, I did not suffer another tension headache for over a month. However, when I again had a headache, I did not rush back for another treatment. It wasn't because of the needles. It was the thought of having to lie still for twenty minutes. Perhaps I could have avoided these if I had laid down or engaged in a daily meditation. However, despite ingesting the contents of those opaque jars, my liver function tests continued to rise, albeit not steadily, until their values had tripled and I was instructed to stop the Casodex. So I did, and I also admit that I stopped the herbs. I was apprehensive now that I wouldn't get a complete anti-androgen effect from the Lupron alone, although my doctors assured me that there was no evidence to justify the fear.

Indeed, my PSA, which had peaked at a value of 6.1 just before the biopsy, fell steadily under the influence of the LHRH agonist/antagonist. By November, just under a month following my first injection, it measured 0.8. By mid-December, shortly after stopping the Casodex, the PSA measured less than 0.1. And by February, it measured 0.06. The Canadian reports had correlated disease regression with the rapidity and depth of fall of the PSA. This seemed like good news, but I was afraid to feel encouraged. One wants to throw the book at cancer and squeeze the last therapeutic drop out of the sponge. Things were looking good, but I had already had sufficient unexpected turns and bad surprises that I couldn't feel confident I would lick this problem.

Then there was the episode in Hawaii. My partner and I had planned a vacation at the end of December, and it seemed like a good idea to go before embarking on radiation. I had not fixed a date to begin radiation, and some of those close to me worried that I might postpone indefinitely. I, for my part, simply wanted to continue comfortably past the lowest PSA I could obtain. The Canadian paper had suggested this nadir most often occurred after 6 to 9 months of hormonal treatment. There was a bit of tension over this plan, since I would not commit to a definite date for the beginning of radiation. Our trip was planned for ten days. The first five of these were characteristically idyllic despite the tension, life at the ocean conveying a sense of timelessness and beauty whose little miracles could be realized simply by sticking one's head under the surface of the water. My little fishy friends, we used to call them. The sun warmed and soothed my body. Fruit tasted great, its from-the-tree freshness so different from the supermarket variety. I felt removed from the cancer, simply a guy in tropical paradise. As I sipped my wine by the sea, I could almost forget I had cancer. It was not to be.

On the fifth day of our trip, I suddenly noticed a walnut-sized lump in my left armpit. Initially, I did not tell my partner. Not only did I not want to rain on our parade, but I knew this ought not to be cancer. I was on hormones. The PSA was low and falling. Prostate cancer typically metastasizes to bone first, then brain and other organs, but the armpit would be bizarre. Yet strange things tend to happen to doctors-turned-patients, and there it was, an unexplained fact in the flesh. My tension showed, my headaches returned. I broke down and told her. Should I call my doctor? Let's just wait a few days, we reasoned, especially since there was no rush to do anything here in the tropics. We went out to dinner, and I did my best to talk about other things. I tried to enjoy the last five days and intermittently pulled it off.

We heard Willie Nelson perform together with his sister and with Kris Kristofferson. We had a good time, except for the unpleasant habit I developed of reexamining my lump many times during the course of each day, sometimes openly and sometimes surreptitiously. I kept hoping it would disappear, in which case I could invoke some bug bite and local reaction. But it did not go away. The only encouraging change was a slight reduction in size during the days I was observing its evolution.

I concluded it must be a lipoma, a benign fat tumor, unrelated to the prostate cancer. It seemed that I had read once of lipomas in relation to changing hormonal milieu, but I might have been making the whole thing up and was never able to document a known relationship. My father had developed a lipoma of the large intestine in his mid-fifties. Ironically, he was thought to have cancer going into surgery, and the diagnosis of a benign tumor in his case was cause for surprise and celebration. We didn't have CT scans or colonoscopy then. Upon our return, I saw my internist, and he agreed that it was likely a lipoma. He was content to leave it alone if I was comfortable with that. Once again, I declined surgery. My lump remains, but it has continued to grow smaller and less well-defined following the cessation of hormonal therapy. I was able to grab the thing and move it around under my skin when I first discovered it. Now I can barely locate it.

Did I have side effects from the Lupron injections? You bet I did, but I was only aware of some of them. I first noted some breast tenderness a few weeks into treatment. It wasn't bad. My biggest fear was that I would grow breasts. That did not happen. To this day, I remain less than an A cup. Any increase in appetite was offset by the negative effects of generalized worry, so I did not gain much weight. My skin seemed to become smoother, a benefit, perhaps, especially in the shaving department. Initially, I sported a full beard, so the difference was hardly noticeable. At the end of my treatment, however, I shed both hair and age, down to a goatee to attain a contemporary look. Shaving was unexpectedly easy, which I attributed to years of not doing so. But many months later, when I was off all therapy including anti-androgens, the whisker challenges returned. I surmised I had enjoyed yet another testosterone effect. My pubic hair thinned. The hair on top of my head did not fall out in clumps, perhaps due to my continuing finestride, which is also prescribed to prevent hair loss due to male-pattern balding.

Since I was not a great athlete before I developed cancer, I did not notice any major loss of muscle strength, another known complication of hormone therapy. I continued to swim twice a week, as I have done for some time, resigned and dedicated to the boredom of maintaining fitness. Perhaps I grew short of breath more quickly than usual. In any event, I was still able to climb the forty-five steps to my front door with relative ease, even when burdened with bags of groceries.

The hardest loss was that of sex drive. The mind and eye continued to work perfectly well. My fantasy world could still be aroused, but little else responded. It is not as though one wakes up one day to find all interest gone. The effect is more gradual and always clouded by overriding anxieties. Fear and worry can affect sexual function, as we all know. But the day inevitably came when I suddenly realized I was simply not the same man I used to be in the man category. Since my partner had similar reasons for reduced sexual interest (due to her treatment for cancer of the endometrium), there wasn't much of an issue. She told me more than once that this was more a man's worry than a woman's. Nevertheless, it seems inevitable that a certain element of loss and shame creeps in when a guy experiences loss of potency. Watching romantic movies where passion and performance always attain Hollywood perfection made the lack seem intolerable. Acts that used to arouse a trigger response in the past now felt no more sexual than a back rub. In fact, they became vaguely annoying. Imagine something previously so pleasurable that men do outrageous and foolish things to obtain it even just for a few minutes, becoming an irritant.

This fact of treatment would be enough to depress anyone. But blocking testosterone can in itself produce depression. I had no idea that I was depressed. I knew I was frightened and worried about the success, cost, and side effects of my cancer treatment. Who wouldn't be worried about that? I continued to smile at work and at home, I thought. I socialized with others, continued to visit my aged mother, ate dinner, watched TV, read books. It was at home that my partner pointed out to me, sometimes in jest and other times in earnest, that my verbal response to almost anything tended to be pessimistic or negative. The low level constant depression got to be somewhat amusing because I was completely unaware of it and my responses seemed to make sense and reflect logic more than mood. I am sure this aura of negativity was no fun for my partner. However, the therapist I saw for support found me appropriate and did not recommend antidepressants, so how bad could it have been? For others, much worse, I understand. Depression from androgen blockade can be clinically significant, even to the point of having to stop treatment. I am told I was more irritable and touchy at home. Was that because of the treatment or because both of us had bad medical problems? Was it due to frustration, my being doubted by physicians and family members? Who knows? What is striking to me even now is that I honestly thought my behavior was completely normal and unaffected by the hormones! This discrepancy remains truly shocking, to think that I was so "under the influence" that I didn't notice, and if someone had confronted me at the time I might have hotly denied that I had changed.

So how did I decide on the total duration of hormone treatment? I did not have much guidance from my physicians. As you may recall, some were doubtful I would derive any benefit beyond shrinking the tumor, which occurs after a couple of months. Others advocated years of hormone treatment without a great deal of data to show significant long-term benefits. The Vancouver group seemed to favor eight to twelve months depending on what was happening with the PSA. My friends and family were increasingly uncomfortable with what they feared might be endless procrastination on my part. In the end time and circumstances provided the answer.

My partner and I had planned a short vacation to Sweden in July. For her, the primary purpose of the trip was to attend a conference in her field. For me, it was to mark the end of my treatment, and in particular, the trip was to be a little reward, a goal to celebrate reaching the endpoint. Tired of pressure to proceed and feeling a bit down from the hormones, I simply worked backwards from the trip, calculating the time required for radiation therapy and seed implantation, and including what I envisioned to be a generous rest period in between. I estimated a four week recovery period for the last step and confirmed that it was reasonable with my seed implant doctor. I then set an early April date to begin radiation therapy. This schedule would provide a total of seven months' hormone treatment preceding radiation and two additional months during radiation. That gave me a total of nine months, and I felt reasonably comfortable with that number of months because my PSA had dropped to a low point so rapidly. The doubt that remained was mostly due to the funny way in which I had decided. Imagine making a decision about a life-threatening illness based largely on travel plans! But it seemed as good a choice as any, given the lack of data and the way I was beginning to feel.

As this first phase of treatment continued and eventually drew to a close, I reflected on what I had learned first hand about the power and wide-ranging effect of hormones. It shames me to think how men sometimes casually throw that word around or fail to realize the profound impact these substances have on all behavior, both male and female. In the end, I had to respect and acknowledge that hormones, and specifically feminizing hormones, may have acted as my medical life preserver. We guys need to watch what we say.

Chapter Seven

Tattoos and Zaps

When all was said and done, I had chosen to have external beam radiation therapy and radioactive seed implants as combined local therapy. I am still not sure I made the right decision, but it felt like the best choice at the time. It is frightening to think that there might not be a right decision. The experts disagree. The patient is pushed to choose, but lacks objectivity. The whole matter continues to have some of the flavor of choosing one suit among many choices at a department store. The interplay between education, fear, and the wish to preserve important bodily functions is too complex to analyze objectively. While I was still trying to decide, I found I was second-guessing myself every time I encountered someone who made a different choice and seemed to have done well. Or conversely, I was completely unsettled when I heard that someone who had had similar treatment had relapsed or suffered nasty complications.

The next question up for debate was where the radiation beam line should be drawn. During the consultation phase, it had not been entirely clear whether my case called for whole pelvis radiation or the more limited conformal prostate radiation. The conformal technique is a sophisticated one of multiple fields arranged in an arc to deliver a maximum dose to the gland from several angles. Because of the wide arc, the normal surrounding tissues are spared the full brunt of the radiation. By covering a wider field, whole pelvis radiation captures some of the possibly involved lymph nodes in the X-ray beam but at the expense of more normal bladder and rectal tissue. The crap shot of efficacy versus additional toxicity once again had reared its ugly head. I was in a gray zone, one in which some radiation oncologists would suggest conformal while others would advocate whole pelvis radiation. In the end, I chose to limit the external beam to conformal. There had been much discussion prior to my decision, but once I stated my choice, everyone seemed to agree to it without objection.

I had decided to have my radiation treatment at the university medical center. The common thread of advice, namely to find a doctor you trust, is challenging for a physician. As a former pediatric oncologist contemplating the treatment of his own tumor, I found this advice extremely difficult to follow. Although I was out of date and far removed from my area of prior knowledge, I knew the ropes and retained the instincts of my former subspecialty. Bedside manner becomes tentative and prickly during physician-to-physician engagements, especially when the doctor-turned-patient is not much older than the treating doctor. Knowledge often becomes a test of competence, placing the treating doctor in a defensive position in which he or she tries to please or convince with overwhelming data. The process is often strained and highly charged. Many doctors choose to pursue a medical career because they do not entirely trust medical treatment over which they have no control. They aspire to control medically, for the good of others, of course, by attacking illness. Aside from selecting a treatment choice, the doctor-turned-patient cannot control what is happening to him, and this relegates him to an unfamiliar passive role. I was very pleased with the intelligence and knowledge of my radiation oncologist. His reputation seemed deserved. Nevertheless, minor inconsistencies in what he said to me on different occasions loomed like massifs, and I found myself torn between my passive patient role and my skeptical, distrusting doctor self. If open and obvious, this doctoritis does not do the doctor-turned-patient any good, so I did my best to control or hide my doubts. I walked the tightrope of being the good patient, the informed consumer, a partner in my own treatment, and a subjective evaluator of the merits of the therapeutic arguments placed before me. Whew!

Somewhere early in the course of my treatment, I became aware of the fact that I would have to be responsible for my own general physical and psychological well-being while in decision-making limbo, as well as during therapy. I also had a responsibility to look after my own body, to maintain strength as best I could. Other cancer patients had stressed that I should be good to myself, whatever that meant. My officemate had given me a book describing some approaches to cancer patient self-kindness, and a hematology colleague had suggested the name of a psychiatrist he had found helpful during a personal medical crisis.

As your typically driven, active pediatrician, I wondered what I would modify about myself and my lifestyle and how I would do it? Would I wait until I was tired before changing my schedule? Would I seek preventive psychotherapy, anticipating inevitable depression, or was this an act of self-indulgence and narcissism? Why fix it if it ain't broke? Why bow to the assumption that all cancer patients become hurt and maimed during their treatment, impaired to the point of requiring help? If I was doing battle with cancer, was it not better to enter the process feeling self-reliant as opposed to dependent on external support?

I did not formulate a conscious plan. Instead, I tried to put certain reality checks in place to tweak my customary patterns when necessary to help me strike a balance between continuing normality and paying attention to my new and changing needs. I entered into treatment as most people do, with a full life, routines, preferences, and obligations. At first, the demands of treatment were minor, their impact hard to gauge. I was receiving shots and taking medicine. Big deal. Nevertheless, I began working on habitual patterns in anticipation of the stresses to come. I instituted an early morning walk at least several days a week. I thought this could serve a number of purposes. First, it would be a relaxing way to begin my day with some mild exercise. I knew that the hormone injections could weaken some joints, notably the hips. Walking would be a good way to maintain the strength of the muscles surrounding my hips, knees, and ankles. Second, healthy exercise would hopefully frame the upcoming day in a positive light. Third, walking exercise could be meditative. In fact, I sometimes listened to tapes as I walked, while other times I simply concentrated on walking briskly, noting the landmarks of my chosen route—about a half a mile, up and down the hilly streets near my house. Occasionally I met a neighbor walking her dog. It was a good beginning that eventually dissipated when bad weather set in, and it came to a complete halt after my seeding.

Although I discontinued the walk, I maintained my other adopted form of exercise, swimming. I am not athletic by desire or inner drive. I chose to swim and had to work at it to overcome inertia. I had joined the YMCA and went to the pool twice a week. It was my practice to do twenty laps. I counted them, not because I was compulsive, but rather because I knew I would begin to cheat if I wasn't keeping a numerical check. During my treatment, I added a few Hebrew liturgical phrases, four word groupings mostly taken from psalms, phrases that would correspond to the strokes between breaths. By following a sequence of these phrases, I could count laps without keeping track of numbers while deriving a mantra-like meditation effect from the swimming. Let's face it, swimming is boring, at least for me. I found this routine to be both satisfying and relaxing. An immediate reward in the hot tub and sauna provided further incentive. Swimming has continued to be my source of exercise and physical relaxation long after the end of my treatment.

I also tried a more formal approach to meditation. Our hospital offered a discounted meditation course to harassed doctors. The grabber was a 30 percent discount on the rather hefty course fee, and, even more importantly, CME credits. These credits are continuing medical education points that doctors in active practice need to generate annually to maintain hospital privileges. In some ways the courses are a racket. They tend to be held in nice places to attract a large number of participants. Some are held in vacation spots like Hawaii to attract family as well as medical participants. A good number of CME courses are accompanied by after-course travel adventures. Most CME courses are informative and they do serve an educational purpose. However, offering CME credits for an eight-week meditation course seemed a bit excessive, although it was tailor-made for my needs, and I was not about to look a gift horse in the mouth. Or so I thought.

I signed up weeks in advance, paid my money, and was actually looking forward to the course as an opportunity to acquire a new method of relaxation. I planned my on-call obligations and chose a radiation time slot with the meditation course in mind. It seemed a little peculiar that attendance requirements were so stringent; the penalty for missing sessions included loss of the hospital's financial contribution and loss of the CME credits. When I told the instructor about my situation, he reassured me that he would be both understanding and accommodating. I bought the required book in advance and arrived early for my first night of meditation, actually an orientation meeting for course participants. The group was small. We introduced ourselves, AA style, sitting in a circle, heard a bit about the course and how it would proceed, were shown the book and the tapes, and were told about an extensive homework requirement. I began to feel a little tense. Sure, the homework was to be meditation, but emphasis was on the seriousness and absolute necessity of the extracurricular time commitment. Toward the close of orientation, we were shown the small cymbals used to signal the beginning and end of a meditation session. Why did this seem stylized and rigid? I hung in there. Our instructor then calmly informed us that there were insufficient people attending that night of the week to conduct the in-class exercises. Therefore, there would not be a class on that weeknight, and people would need to choose one of the other two available times to join a larger group. I was furious and did not contain my anger. Very non-Buddhist. No, I said, I could not change all my on-call nights at the last minute for an eight-week stint. No, I could not change my radiation time slot. He maintained his calm. No matter how I objected or pleaded, he maintained his calm. He kept inviting me to change my life. What a pity, he exclaimed calmly, and how he sympathized, calmly, and how he understood that I, especially, was in need of his stress reduction course because of the cancer, calmly, but there was no way he could conduct this class except in the fashion to which he was accustomed. My meditation experience thus came to a crashing halt. I received a full refund and the instructor calmly offered to lend me his copy of the book, the one I had already bought along with a meditation tape. I tried the tape, but found that just hearing the instructor's soothing voice reawakened all the anger I had experienced and further agitated me with its ever-present calmness.

Looking back on this episode, I wonder whether I would have been so riled up if I didn't have cancer. Someone has to be the fall guy for the anger we really feel about having been stricken. But at the time I could only ask, how could he be so unmoved? Did this person, who should represent sensitivity-in-action, not care at all? I was appalled by what I perceived as unreasonable rigidity in the face of my illness. How dare he compare the urgency of my need against any petty standard he might have. I was being discounted. Nothing about his bland expression of concern, accompanied by what seemed to be studied and acquired placidity, placated my fury. I had come for tension reduction and experienced stress enhancement. Considering the trouble I had gone through to be free to take this class, I saw no more than simple intransigence, or, even worse, possible laziness. Clearly, I would have to find another method of meditation. Perhaps my impatient personality did not lend itself to meditation practices at all.

For my birthday, about a month later, a dear friend gave me a precious gift. She bought me an hour with her personal yoga instructor, a lesson to be given in my home. I made the arrangements and was visited by a kind, practiced woman who guided me through a variety of restorative, gentle contortions. I stretched muscles I never knew I possessed. We worked from the book I had bought for the meditation course, and she pointed out sequences that she thought I would find helpful. I had bought a mat for the exercises and truly enjoyed the session and was relaxed by its close. I was pretty sore the next day. Clearly a step in the right direction, I thought. I followed up a few times on my own, but did not continue with lessons and did not join a yoga group. Groups are not my thing. The mat hangs in the closet under the shelf that is home to my MRI.

Meanwhile, I clung to my obligations. I maintained my schedule at the office. I visited my aged mother twice a week. I helped out at home. I spoke with my daughter and guided her when asked. I helped with the groceries. I remained on my synagogue's Board of Directors. One might feel that obligations are a strain not to be continued during cancer treatment, and, depending on the fatigue and stress factor, this may indeed be true. However, I derived comfort and strength from being needed. Obligations frame my daily life, and they provided me with a sense of continuity throughout my treatment period. Perhaps I was a bit excessive at the expense of relaxation, but the total contribution was one I still feel to have been positive. One should never feel beleaguered by obligations while receiving treatment for cancer. But if they add to a sense of mastery while that treatment is underway, more power to you I say. The hard part is judging what is too much, before it really is too much.

I undertook creative projects. I began writing, casually at first, jotting down reactions, ideas, random thoughts and reflections. An article had appeared in a leading medical journal presenting data showing that keeping a journal could have a positive impact on chronic illness. As my treatment progressed, I found I had more to say, both to myself and potentially to others. Those random records, not quite a journal or diary, eventually germinated and gelled into this book.

I also added a new element of innovation to my professional work, another creative effort, about the time of my therapy. I had long been interested in teaching parents of toddlers and older children how to view their kids' eardrums. The pediatric world had just awakened to the hazards of freely dispensed antibiotics, so the time was right to act on my interest. I wanted to develop a research project in the pediatric practice setting, one that would test the feasibility of parents excluding the diagnosis of ear infection at home. To this end, I took on a student just before my diagnosis was established, and we put the project together. I worked on this despite the cancer, spending hours at the computer, talking with colleagues, obtaining the approval of the hospital's Research Committee and Institutional Review Board. Gone are the days when a doctor could simply try something new in his office. My little project was hotly debated on its merits, attacked, revised, and dissected with respectful skepticism. Since I also sit on one of these committees, I was used to the process and certainly participated in it eagerly when the work of others was being evaluated. But, give me a break! I was just trying to do a little innocuous project in my office! No blood tests. No painful procedures. No big budget. Why all the fuss at a time like this? Eventually, the project did pass and we began the process of selling the idea to other pediatricians. That proved fruitless. We were unable to generate any interest. In fact, there was a surprising amount of resistance, mostly passive. Despite all the obstacles, I think it was enormously helpful to my psyche to be able to invest intellectual energy in a side project such as this one in the midst of my treatment.

My student, then a premedical student, now about to enter medical school, stuck with me, developed and implemented the project, shared the ups and downs that comprised our effort of trying to carry it out, and became a friend and support to me in the process. Her own mother had died of breast cancer, and she still very much mourned her loss, yet she was able to see my need for her company and cheer me on. The ear examination project eventually fizzled for lack of community interest. Not only had it kept me busy, however, it had provided creative distraction. It took my mind off my troubles and changed my perspective. Creative acts also add a sense of forward motion to your life. While you are threatened and vulnerable, you nevertheless are able to add something new to the world, a thought, a product, or an action. It certainly does not need to be a professional project.

It just turned out that way for me. My officemate had taken up poetry and pottery, which she continues to this day. I also sought distraction in music, my other avocation, and I joined a former neighbor of mine in some music lessons, which we were able to continue until I began radiation.

Music, I have come to realize, is my most reliable form of meditation, and I have sought refuge in playing recorder ever since I made this discovery. A life-threatening illness can be the impetus to attend to one's creative self. It draws attention to this oft-buried need and fertilizes its growth into a necessity. I no longer wish to be without music making for any significant length of time. When I play music, I am in another world where I completely express my inner self.

So far, I had patched together a little tripartite self-care program. This was comprised of physical activity, maintaining a balanced set of obligations that preceded the cancer diagnosis, and initiating some new, creative endeavors providing positive distraction. A close, though more passive, ally of creative distraction is entertainment, another tonic for the self. Entertainment, for the most part, is done to you. It can arouse your emotions, help you laugh, or provide distraction. During the winter months, I attended concerts and some movies. I stuck to a local baroque music concert series I had been attending annually for more than fifteen years. There were dinners out, shared with my partner, with or without additional friends. Entertainment that does not require much from you other than engagement is inherently pampering. When you are undergoing cancer treatment, because you may not feel entirely well for a lengthy period of time, any form of pampering can serve as a temporary, but significant antidote. I am also a shameless baseball fan, so with the advent of spring, I resumed watching ballgames. I think very few people would contend that the world hangs in the balance on the merits and achievements of an athlete or a team. Yet we can go nuts over competitive sports. I think it may be because we take on the excellence and power of athletic achievement. Perhaps this is also why we are so moved when an athlete is stricken with debilitating injury or illness. Somehow, watching these strong baseball players competing for ever-greater physical superiority gave me a feeling of inner strength. Furthermore, all sports are ritualized by their rules and carry within their structure the promise of civility and an element of predictability. No one will ever be rewarded for running retrograde from third base to first base. Sure, there have to be surprises, otherwise the whole matter would be dull. But the underpinnings are stabilized by ritual, and I needed overt and covert suggestions of stability throughout my treatment.

I also cared for myself through spiritual practice, or religious ritual. The topic is always touchy, and I do not wish to preach about its virtues or belabor it. In whatever way we recognize the set of qualities we describe as the soul, this part of us also needs attention during cancer treatment. Whether it be meditation, psychotherapy, prayer, attending church, synagogue, temple, or mosque, or whether it be painting, singing, or sculpting carried out with mental awareness, all spiritual practice has at least two factors in common. First, it will be ritualized and repetitive. Second, it will serve to focus the participant's mind so his life and the events occurring to him are placed in some perspective and take on a more neutral aspect. This redirecting of our minds, souls, or human spirit is calming and hopefully uplifting.

I found all these measures to be especially vital as the treatment period ground away for months on end, beginning with the relatively benign hormone therapy and advancing to the more menacing and irreversible radiation and seeds. Spiritual activities may not necessarily achieve control over a process that is beyond our control. But they can give us a sense of ourselves, a positive sense of what we as human beings can do with our lives whether they are currently lived in a state of health or not. These activities, by emphasizing our vitality, can combat depression and anxiety.

Meanwhile, I was about to begin radiation. There exists a potentially depressing, subterranean quality to radiation therapy, much like a descent into the netherworld. First, most facilities are located in hospital basements. This arrangement arises from lead shielding requirements as well as from the weight of the equipment. The location eliminates windows. One is given the sense that something secretive and not-to-be seen is taking place, something that needs to be contained, private, and invisible. The radiation therapy facility may resemble boxes within boxes, a basement labyrinth comprised of a waiting and check-in room, a dressing room, a secondary sex-segregated waiting room, and a treatment room. Each of these chambers is enclosed and stuffy, resembling a catacomb. I felt like I was participating in a live burial, lying down and immobile on the treatment table, strapped down in the deathly silent, innermost box.

The locker rooms are particularly strange, as they mark a transition point between the outside and inside worlds. For me, changing into therapy pajamas meant changing from doctor to patient. Various details began to take on major associations. The radiation therapy lockers have old, flimsy locks, opened and closed by keys attached to small rectangular plastic plates. I noted that in the radiation suite, each man had a signature approach to key placement, either holding the key in his hand or placing it in a shirt pocket, or, most popularly, in a shoe. By contrast, my gym locker looks the same, but it is secured by my combination lock. I have an assigned locker at the gym. I never even thought to use a particular locker at radiation therapy. Why bother for a ten-minute experience? Opening each of the two different lockers reminded me of the other, thus linking a pleasurable association, swimming, with an emotionally painful and threatening one, radiation. It seemed strange that in the hospital locker and changing rooms there was neither the smell of chlorine nor that of post-exercise sweat. There also was no laughter.

Radiation therapy suites tend to be populated by two basic sets of people. First you have the patients, typically wandering around in gowns, partially and periodically revealing various parts of their bodies marked with lines, circles, or crosses. Street clothes sometimes protrude, revealing the individuality of shoes and socks masked by the uniformity of the hospital gown. Then there are staff, technicians, nurses, and doctors, forming an integrated internal unit, often dressed in white or in surgical scrubs, placing and manipulating the patients into various positions at varying times, adjusting heavy equipment, and scurrying in and out of the rooms housing the patients. Machines hum and fall silent. Others creak and groan. Just to tweak the anxiety button some, the sounds are not uniform and leave you guessing when the radiation beam is on and when it is off. Lights go on and off, identifying mysterious transitions. You learn the routine after a while, becoming familiar with signals of anticipation.

Preparation for radiation therapy largely involves a series of targeting X rays and CT scans, defining the radiation beam fields, followed by the tattoo session. The measurements are very sophisticated, computerized, exact, but the external manifestation of what is going on can be gross and shifting. At various intervals, the purple magic marker lines are repositioned, and they may not appear symmetrical. One begins to question their accuracy, especially when Monday's technician is not the same as Friday's. I was instructed not to scrub them off, a seemingly simple assignment. Yet one day, when I was inattentive, I dried myself vigorously after a shower and pretty much destroyed a mark. I was mortified and embarrassed, but the tech simply took a few more films and drew it on again, in a slightly different place, of course. The episode sent me back to my radiation oncologist for reassurance, and he said he would personally check the scout films against my markings. What was most unnerving was that despite my knowledge of what comprised a radiation dose, each X-ray film seemed like a window of accumulating danger. I couldn't escape the notion that X rays are bad for you. The knowledge that the fields and doses are a computerized product lends an aura of precision and accuracy that may be overstated. All radiation comes with scatter. Every normal cell cannot be completely shielded from the beam. The human factor has not been removed from the planning and execution of the treatment ports; the aim, if you will, and the shots delivered against the cancer are still fired by an imperfect human being.

What is most eerie about all of this is that nothing hurts and there are moments of protracted quiet and solitude during which nothing seems to be happening, interludes providing curious comfort and a sense of security, moments suggesting peace and shelter during which you can imagine lying on a lawn or in a canoe, comfy and safe.

One tries to forget that these X rays, which most of us have assiduously avoided during our healthy periods, are burning and destroying body cells, both cancerous and noncancerous, each time the machine whirs and the lights blink. Whether radiation side effects are minimal or severe, and even knowing that alternatives also destroy or remove healthy tissues, there remains a sense of self-destruction, a nagging question as to whether the gain is indeed going to be worth the damage done. Medicinal treatment defies our intuition, because reason tells us it is good to build and bad to destroy. The most common exception to this notion is that of battle against an enemy, where it is good to destroy, so we enlist our bodies and our minds in the mother of all fights to lick cancer, the bad guy. The battle of radiation therapy becomes a war of attrition, in which survival of good cells and bad cells are pitted against each other every time we are zapped.

In the case of prostate cancer, three tattoo dots are placed, one in the pubic area, and one on each hip. Tattoos sting for a second or two. What really hurts is the thought of being marked permanently and in a manner and location that you will remember for the rest of your life. The magic marker lines and crosses drawn near or over the tattoos, lines that make up the last and final alignment, are more obvious and glaring, but are also readily removable. For five weeks I wondered whether anyone in the gym shower would notice, casts glances, or ask about these marks. I never sensed that anyone noticed, this despite my being acutely self-conscious about them and covering up with a towel right after

a shower. I suppose keeping one's eyes to oneself is part of locker room etiquette. We are also geared to see what we expect, so
no one showering after a swim is likely to think of radiation therapy unless they are a physician or a fellow patient. Despite the
smattering of a variety of large and small artistic tattoos on other
bodies, tattoos designed to be noticed, my temporary body artistry
remained a very private affair.

To enter the radiation room is to be submissive. You lie on
the hard table and feel its unwillingness to yield as it blocks any
escape from the beam above. Your feet are bound, your legs
encased in a mold specially constructed to fit the contours of your
body. You are instructed not to help while cheerful technicians
move your lower half, pulling and tugging you into position by
yanking on the sheet beneath you. The marks drawn on your
body are targeted as though you are the objective of some of
Gulliver's little gunners. Then, with a friendly wave, the technicians leave you, bound and secured, alone with the machine.

During the moments of silence preceding radiation, I sometimes listened to the piped music, sometimes stared at the X-ray
unit, and sometimes tried to think about something or somewhere
else. There were moments of anxiety and low-level panic. What
was I doing there? Where was everybody? Was the X-ray machine
aimed right? Could I feel the beam or was I imagining it? Initially,
I was so stiff lying on the table, so tense, so afraid to breathe, that
I think I strained some muscles and gave myself hip and back
pain. I felt my skin itching where my body was marked. Then,
as the days and weeks went on, these sensations subsided and
radiation became routine, as everything eventually does. I entered
into this midday rhythm with some equanimity, a strange hiatus

separating morning and afternoon. This routine became a Monday through Friday bracket, lasting five weeks. The weekend rest periods conveniently have a physiologic justification. Some tissue recovery time actually aids the process of radiation therapy. I would close up pediatric shop an hour before noon, get in my car, turn on the radio, mixing music with traffic news reports, zip into the city, park at the university medical center, and make my way to radiation therapy. Since it was lunchtime, I got to see lots of "normal" people and imagine myself one of them.

Approximately half a dozen of us patients hovered around the same treatment period, which I began to think of as the lunchtime radiation hour. There was overlap and dropout as people started or ended on differing schedules. Nevertheless, a kind of camaraderie developed among the assembled, and we exchanged stories and opinions during variably brief or protracted waiting periods. Except for the purpose of our convocation, we could have been seen as a fabulous social mix, a group of people who ordinarily would not meet, but suddenly and unpredictably were thrown together. It reminded me of films in which passengers on a voyage fall into a situation of shared isolation, such as being marooned on an island, an imposed grouping that forces them to relate to each other and help one another. We made up the following colorful array: There was a semi-retired fifty-six year-old ER doc, a fatalist whose father had died of prostate cancer. We had an audiologist, retired, from Montana. This man had just undergone a skull biopsy to check a suspicious area and he joined us wearing a stocking bandage wound around his head. Our internist, a man who had already undergone years of treatment, sought refuge in knowledge and logic. We had a retired carpenter who had previously undergone heart angioplasty and walked 5 miles a day to maintain his health. We had a man who could tell us stories about his career in pest control. And then we were joined by an accountant who commuted a fair distance to radiation therapy, a cheerful man always carrying around his gym bag, a man who was having to receive radiation following surgery. He was the only man who actually carried his valuables with him as advised by signs in the locker room. Another guy, conversant in old Anglo-Saxon was a Beowulf buff. Toward the end of my treatment, an Asian man, perhaps Vietnamese, who didn't say much, joined us. We must all have been wondering about him, because prostate cancer is said to be relatively rare among Asians. It was quite a group of guys, all with the same problem, all taking what they could from the comfort of company.

Also present in the waiting room were various men with other conditions, bearing different marks, having different parts of their bodies exposed, some carrying chemo infusion setups. It is a hard thing to admit, but I suspect some distancing took place between the prostate guys and the "others." It is the kind of distancing that occurs when you hope and pray that yours is a curable kind of cancer. Conversely, I imagined that some of these other men thought us lucky, as we sat in our pajama bottoms and tried to make light conversation. Once we talked about movies. We could have been at a cocktail party except for the purpose of our convocation and our peculiar dress.

The conversation was largely disjointed. Few topics carried over from one day to the next. The talk moved in and out of discussions about prostate cancer according to the comfort level and interest of those present at the time. Some men were more sensitive than others in assessing the potential impact of their words. The three of us who were doctors were asked medical questions, despite our personal vulnerability and uncertainty. Some questions were general, and answering them was familiar and comforting. Other questions were close to the bone, even unwittingly challenging, such as "Why did you choose X" or "Why didn't you do Y?" This was always unsettling. We heard bits and pieces of each other's lives. No one spoke of side effects. Either none were experienced, or the experiences were not readily shared. Some tales were richly entertaining, such as the story about a strict blackout order at a site in North Africa during World War II accompanying a secret meeting between Roosevelt and Churchill, during which a buddy of the guy telling the story almost shot Churchill when he thoughtlessly lit a cigar. Hearing World War II stories brought home my relative youth within this group.

One by one we were called to the X-ray machine. The system used to determine the order of treatments seemed archaic. There was a small basket on the check-in counter in the waiting room. As people arrived, they wrote their name and the number of their X-ray machine on a scrap of paper provided for this purpose, and deposited the slip in the basket. Thereafter, each of us made his way to the inner waiting room by way of the changing room. If someone scheduled ahead of you was late and your name was in the basket, you might get called early. If everyone was present, the schedule was followed. The machine sometimes broke down or was afflicted with a problem, causing a potentially long wait. Fortunately, I was never delayed more than an hour. The chances of experiencing a long delay increased for those undergoing eight weeks of radiation as opposed to my five.

The X-ray unit tracks an unwanted radiation embrace. The beam's housing encircles you as it moves from left to right. It stops four or seven times as it traverses its arc, depending on the type of radiation you are receiving. When it comes to radiation therapy, most doctors might as well be lay people. If you want to understand what is going on, you need to be a bit of a physicist. I had sent patients to radiation therapy for years without knowing much about the particulars. The machine hums or buzzes when it is turned on. You feel nothing. You don't really know what is going on when, except on the basis of what you hear, much like an isolated prisoner who can only listen to find out what is happening outside his cell. The beam comes on as an interruption of the regular electrical hum. It can be discerned by a change in pitch of the hum, or, in other positions, by a quiet, rapid rat-a-tat sound. The unit moves and stops, sometimes seeming to groan and complain a bit about being forced to change position. In a seven-field technique, it turns off both midway and at the end. You begin to experience the process as three plus four separate events. As a doctor, you might think about what lies in the anatomic path of each beam position. Although you are essentially immobilized from the waist down, there is a tendency to hold your breath when you think the beam is on. I felt I had to make a conscious effort not to stiffen my muscles, as though to prevent even the slightest motion, to avoid inducing any inaccuracy while under the beam. This was patently ridiculous, of course.

There is a strange silence and sense of being alone while you are with the machine. I had some very anxious moments which came as a surprise to me, since I knew intellectually that the actual radiation exposure caused no discomfort. But I also knew that

the beam's effect was not benign. For a while, I became patho-
logically anxious and a little light-headed, and I felt my heart
beating hard during the treatment period. While feeling no pain,
I thought about the ultimate source of the X-ray beam travers-
ing my body. I contemplated its scientific source. I also considered the phenomenon of cosmic radiation, which is present
throughout the universe. Thus, a powerful, indirectly perceived,
universal force, radiation, was being harnessed to serve my individual need, redirected toward an inconsequential minute event
in the universe. It all seemed quite remarkable and awesome.

When I told a friend who also had cancer about my anxiety
under the beam, she recalled having the same experience and told
me she began to think of X rays as the healing power of God. She
had tried to perceive this power as an affirmation, a thought
designed to help her make herself well. Think of primordial radiation as bathing the universe with a power we normally do not
notice. Imagine borrowing from this power and using it, much as
Prometheus borrowed fire. When spiritual healers speak of energy, even a skeptic can appreciate the relationship of energy to matter and contemplate the incorporation of radiation energy into our
bodies. We can be damaged or comforted and made to feel well
by other, more familiar, forms of energy such as sunshine, heat, or
rushing water. These can play on our senses, while radiation does
not. I tried to look upon the beam as a cosmic gift emanating from
the divine, possibly to heal me rather than cause me harm.

The end of radiation therapy was almost an anticlimax. Five
weeks pass quickly, if one is pain free. I didn't count days or
therapy sessions until I was near the end. A pleasurable long weekend trip interrupted the treatment time and provided a nice lit-

tle respite as well as a short-term goal. Anticipating even a two day vacation break mid-term, helped the time pass more quickly. A slight miscalculation on the part of the therapists caused a momentary debate among the technicians and radiation oncologists as to my actual last day. It might not make much difference, but a dose is a dose. The fractionation of X-ray treatments over weeks is not an accident, as it takes into account that day-to-day tissue recovery and the cumulative effect of the X-ray beam. On my last day, a Friday, I forgot a gift of cookies despite my wish to thank the staff. I just wanted to get out of there. The mold that had encased my legs was offered to me as a souvenir, but I declined.

I emerged from the hospital basement a free man released from midday confinement. I had some fatigue during the final week, but was relatively well. No urinary irritation, no diarrhea, nothing. I departed, leaving behind the ER doc who had chosen to have all his therapy by external beam radiation, and would have to continue three to four weeks longer. We parted with mutual good luck wishes, the mantra of prostate cancer, our paths diverging, each wondering about the other's decision and future course. I still wonder how he is doing.

There was a planned break between the external beam treatment and seed implantation. It was hard to conceive that things continued to happen in my body during this time without any awareness on my part, that the effect of the radiation was to continue for months and even years. My recovery from external beam radiation seemed instantaneous. I enjoyed the days and nights like a vacation. A couple of experiments to determine whether my sexual apparatus continued to function were successful until the days immediately preceding departure for my seed implants. We prepared for the trip as though it was going to be a short vacation, packed accordingly, and made our way to the airport as we had planned. I did my best to submerge any feelings of anxiety, adopting a piece-of-cake attitude belied by inner turmoil I tried to conceal. The last treatment leg, the invasive one, was suddenly imminent.

Chapter Eight

Sowing Seeds

From everything I read, it appeared that the expertise involved in accurate and successful seed implantation was critical. The timing and nature of seeding were hotly debated. Some physicians implanted seeds first followed by external beam. Others did it the other way around. Some used permanent implants, placed once and left to decay over a number of weeks. Others used temporary implants that were removed after doing their job. Temporary implants might be placed in the prostate at intervals during external beam radiation, and left in the gland for minutes or overnight. There were isotope choices, iodine versus palladium. Here, more than anywhere, there were no facts to guide me to a decision. I had to rely on the reasoning offered by the implanter, and needless to say, everyone I spoke with had very strong, and seemingly reasonable, opinions on the subject.

The investment, both technical and emotional, in a given seed treatment approach is considerable. No wonder each seeder felt certain that his approach was the best one. One person who was well reputed in the field was a former colleague of mine. I decided not to consider his program because he was located in the Midwest and because his technique would require two seeding procedures in the dead of winter. What a way to make a decision. My local person felt too close. I did not feel comfortable being treated at my own hospital. Others felt too far. In the end, I chose to go to Seattle primarily because the group there had the most implant experience and was still sufficiently regional so as to not impose the additional strain of lengthy travel.

My scientist friend, whose treatment preceded mine by a few months, had also chosen to have seed implantation in Seattle rather than locally. He too had admitted that his was more an emotional decision buttressed by the rationale of published experience. I found myself following his footsteps in this regard, much like a navigator in flight might adjust his flight plan on the basis of reports offered by the pilot of the plane flying ahead of him.

In addition, the person in Seattle who eventually was to seed my prostate was the first doctor I had spoken to after my MRI. He had been very helpful and comforting when I was terrified, anticipating a positive biopsy. That bond can be very strong when it comes time to choose who will poke you. I had called him shortly after getting the biopsy pathology report, before I actually met with any consultants. He had been enormously reassuring, low key, complimentary about the experts in my geographic area, yet subtly open and inviting about his own implant setup. As I spoke with him, it became obvious that seed implantation was an especially facile routine for him. Here was a person, I thought, who was modest despite being self-assured. That was encouraging.

I had completed a two-week rest period following external beam radiation, and I was feeling relatively good. I wasn't overly fatigued and suffered no discomfort or urinary or bowel side effects. I had suppressed most of the seed horror stories I had heard, choosing instead to remember the examples of men who had had no difficulty. I spoke with the father of a close friend of mine, a physician now in his eighties, who had just had seeds, and he described short-term discomfort, followed by rapid resumption of normal activities. In short, I was primed for a lark.

Lest I be too nonchalant, this was a procedure that would involve spinal anesthesia. People experience a vast range of anticipation and worry when threatened by anything invasive. Some men and women are relatively undisturbed by this. I have known people who had little anxiety due to a strong faith in God, and others, agnostics or atheists, who were simply cavalier about fate when faced with the inevitability of illness, pain, and death. Others like me seem to be anxious about anything that is done to their body. The degree of anxiety I experienced would govern my need for control. The more I worried, the more I needed to control and the more I believed that perhaps I could somehow influence the process and the outcome. I knew the chance of serious complications was very low but I was tense about it nevertheless, and this hurdle occupied my mind as my partner and I flew the short hop to Seattle. The fear of complications colored my thinking as I slipped into a mood of nervous anticipation.

After our initial phone contact, I had two face-to-face contacts with my implant physician prior to the actual seeding. The first, a consultation, had come early in my diagnosis, when I was just beginning hormone treatment, before I had made the decision to have seeds. On that trip, I heard about the nuts and bolts of his operation, very slick and professional, and I toured the setting where this group of physicians did their work, which consisted entirely of seed implantation. The scope of the facility was impressive and inspired confidence. I was reminded of the difference between a pediatric floor in a general hospital and a hospital entirely devoted to the care of children. During my meeting with the physician who was to do the procedure, the advantages of implantation over surgery were once again laid out for me. The data were reviewed. I received an encouraging prognosis, together with a very strong message that my cancer had likely spread beyond the capsule of the prostate gland. No great surprise, I guess, that his vote was strongly for external beam radiation plus seed implantation.

The consultation, with my permission, was carried out in the presence of a doctor-in-training, a young physician who had traveled to Seattle to learn about seed implantation. I love students and enjoy teaching in my own practice. Although I immediately said yes, I felt a bit invaded by having become a "teaching case," and I drew the line when it came to the obligatory rectal examination. There was going to be only one of those, and it was to be done by my physician. I suppose it was educational that this student saw how it was to deal with a physician-turned-patient. Every word had to be measured and justified by data.

The second trip to Seattle came before external beam radiation. This was for a so-called "volume study" where an ultrasound examination measures the prostate in order to plan the details of seed implantation. It was in this planning, computerized and exacting, where the experience of the Seattle group was most likely to be beneficial. The meticulousness of the advance planning and the skill with which the plan is executed are paramount. This is not a casual procedure that should be undertaken just anywhere.

Circumstances gave me the luxury of deciding between having seeds implanted locally or traveling to "mecca." It was a difficult decision. I had a choice among three well-qualified and personable people. The decision came down to criteria I knew to be somewhat weak. It is true that experience, the number of procedures performed, was an important factor, but that criterion did not help me. These three individuals were trained in the same fashion. They all knew and respected each other. None would do me the favor of dumping on the other. In fact each gave me to understand that any one of the three would do an acceptable job. I was tortured by this decision, wishing to make it on rational grounds but being continuously thrown back on soft, intuitive factors. To this day, I am not entirely sure I know what triggered my final decision, beyond the deadlines that confronted me. There was a long period during which I remained undecided, much to the consternation of my partner. She saw my vacillation as torture heaped upon misery. It was hard to explain to a layperson how a physician could be so indecisive about a medical decision, especially a person used to making definitive and decisive determinations daily in the course of pediatric practice.

Much of these scenarios coursed through my mind as we landed in Seattle. However, part of me behaved as though we were on vacation. I had lived in Seattle and remained familiar with the city. I had completed part of my pediatric training in Seattle, notably, a fellowship in pediatric hematology and oncology. I derived some comfort from my having a history here. But there was also the discomfort of being an older patient in a realm where I previously had identified myself as an up-and-coming young physician. I could not escape the passage of time, much like a traveler who returns to places where he spent part of his youth, only to find that what once appealed, was no longer attractive, and what was once easy was now difficult. On our previous trips to Seattle, we had managed to combine the unfortunate business with pleasure. This time, the sense of pleasure was missing entirely. I had relinquished any last vestige of control by not renting a car. My partner and I took the Airporter to its downtown destination. We could have taken a cab from there. Instead, we chose to walk the few blocks to our hotel, a comfortable older establishment that offered a room discount to patients of the institute. The walk was all uphill, a physical metaphor for the climb upon which I had embarked. I was in good shape and felt relatively well physically. In my mind, I was already playing the "tomorrow at this time . . . " game and trying to maintain an air of confidence.

Before the plane landed, I took a bowel prep, magnesium citrate, to clear out my intestines in preparation for the next day's seeding procedure. Stool in the lower large intestines and rectum can distort the shape and position of the prostate gland, and, if it performs an untimely exit, can contaminate the operative field. Therefore, it must be got rid of. Little did I know what was in store for me as we prepared to take a short walk downtown to get some fresh air.

I made it about three blocks down the hill from the hotel. Then I got one of those subtle physical signals that periodically remind us that our minds are not in complete control of our bodies. I cannot describe or even recall the feeling. I only knew without question that it was time to turn around. I bounded back up the hill and headed straight to the bathroom, just barely in time. For the next four to five hours, I had constant cramps of a severity I had not experienced since being afflicted with food poisoning in Turkey some twenty years ago. The pain, sweating, and shaking that accompanied this prep were close to unbearable. I can admit now that I had cheated on the magnesium citrate, only taking about half of the prescribed amount. On some level, I must have known what could happen. Had someone offered me general anesthesia at that point, I might have taken it. Imagine being so wiped out by a potion that precedes the Big Event, that the latter is virtually forgotten. All I could do was wonder when this agony would end. It did end, of course, and, as manifestation of yet another miracle of human recovery, I was able to joke about the experience the next day. However, the ultimate indecency was caloric. I was not to eat solid food after midnight, NPO (or null par orum, in medical parlance). Because my surgery was to be at noon, I was limited to clear liquids the next morning. Therefore, the combination of bowel cleansing plus NPO felt like a crash diet completed before stressful exercise, and I entered the seeding procedure feeling weak and hungry, deprived of basic sustenance. These are some of the preparatory procedures we hold so necessary for the safety and success of a medical undertaking. At the same time, they are disturbingly counterintuitive. The part of our physical core that lacks medical sophistication would like to have had a T-bone steak and a good night's sleep before such a procedure. Keeping us hail and hearty would seem more appropriate. About an hour before the seeding, I walked the two blocks to the hospital check-in, feeling nervous but strangely confident. I was sure that the whole thing would be behind me before dinner.

Check-in once again achieved that instant emotional transformation from doctor to patient with which I had unhappily become so familiar. I negotiated a series of steps past the blood draw and into the outpatient pre-op waiting room. I don't recall reading magazines. Perhaps I spoke with my partner. I undoubtedly looked around the waiting room trying to assess what the others were in for as a means of retaining my medical edge over mere mortals. It was not long before an anesthesiologist appeared and introduced himself to me, ahead of schedule. Our talk was brief. He knew that I understood medical procedures, and, in immediate mutual comprehension, spared me the usual litany of potential complications of having a spinal. I signed the papers and we were ready to go. It is part of the anesthesiologist's job to walk the patient down to the operating room. It is a strange ritual dictated by circumstance. I think most any patient would prefer to transition from normalcy to surgery in the comfort of a nice room, perhaps in the company of a friend, and listening to music, then wake up refreshed with the whole thing behind him. Alas, we must be fully conscious and place ourselves on the operating table, the ultimate gesture of volition. So that is what I did. I took leave of my partner, and the anesthesiologist and I walked down the aisle. Out of context, we might have looked like an odd couple, the guys in blue taking a stroll.

I was met by a cheerful crowd, music going, my operating seeder ready with the engine running, his entourage poised to do his bidding. Small wonder that such rooms are called operating theaters in Britain! Here was The Show. I was The Act of the Hour, but my role was as prop, not the talent.

I was introduced to the urologist of the day, who would place the catheter into my bladder and assist during the procedure. The catheter was necessary both to locate the bladder and the prostate in relation to it. My bladder also had to remain empty by being drained of urine. An ultrasound probe would be placed into my rectum to delineate it as well as to provide images of the prostate. Pinned between the two, deep inside my paralyzed body, the prostate gland was to remain stationary like a dartboard before the darts.

While all of this may sound intimidating, I was strangely comfortable with it. We are very much at ease in familiar surroundings, and the operating room with all of its machinery, lights, and instrument trays was a part of my day-to-day medical life. The roles in that chamber were emotionally interchangeable. Except for my being the one on the table, the whole scene might have been a snapshot taken of me at work attending a Cesarian section. The fluoroscope, the personnel, the sights and sounds of the OR, if anything, were actually reassuring. But I was not given a lot of time to think about it. Unfortunately, I had to be the patient in this picture.

Right away, I was lying on my left side and my back was being cleansed. I barely felt the needle poke, followed by a warm tingling in my buttocks and legs. I had been offered Versed, a medication that reduces anxiety and also induces amnesia. The urologist gave me a "why not?" look and I went for it. I was rolled onto my back, quickly becoming numb from the waist down. The various indecencies penetrating my orifices were placed when I could not feel them. I heard coordinates being shouted out and acknowledged, A1, C2, C3, etc., as I became a Cartesian wonder while feeling nothing more than some detached giddiness. It was all over in about half an hour, punctuated by encouraging words from my seeding surgeon or interventionist or whatever constitutes a proper title for this man who was cheerfully saving me from awful surgery. All was going well, he said. All went well, he said. It was over. The urologist who had placed a catheter into my numb penis went back to look and happily showed me the inside of my bladder on the flouroscope screen. What fun. There I was, my mind alert, not forgetting, able to scratch my nose, and completely detached from the lower half of my body. Only my mind knew I had been poked twenty-five times with long needles that contained over a hundred radioactive pellets. It seemed that the anesthesia was deepening as I was lifted onto a gurney and wheeled from the operating room. Such trips feel strange when you are looking up at a moving ceiling you usually take for granted with daily oblivion. Ceilings are not necessarily interesting, but together with human figures seen from below and culminating in heads shrouded in surgical blues, they constitute an odd visual impression experienced by half a body attached to a floating sensorium. I was awake, but looped.

In the Recovery Room, one enters a series of transition zones, rather like locks of a canal transporting a ship to safe passage from one sea to another. To attain freedom, one has to meet certain criteria determining stability and safety. As I got settled and felt the numbness actually increasing, I thought it might be a long wait. The nurses were terrific and cheerful. I immediately asked to have my partner visit, feeling relieved and high, wishing to share my having survived. But there was this little problem with my blood pressure. It was quite low, and I had to wait for it to rise to a normal level before anyone could visit me. And wait I did, for about an hour. I think I dozed a bit and listened to music, but I'm not sure. All I remember is my amazement at the heavy, wooden burden of my lower body, especially on my left side, which had briefly been in a downward facing position when the anesthetic was first injected.

I say "burden" because there was no feeling in my lower half, and my legs seemed an encumbrance. I could run my hands down my back toward my buttocks and feel the exact level where paralyzed nerves had been tricked into temporary absence of sensation. I pressed inward, noting the slight give of my skin, now lacking in all feedback, both pleasurable and irritating. I could not have been caressed, tickled, teased, or hurt below the belt, but just lay there, waiting, like a block of wood set aside for a project. I did notice that there was a large pad between my legs. This brought about bizarre associations, since most of my experience with patients recovering from spinals was with postpartum mothers who had had epidurals for delivery. Their pads were for the bleeding that followed vaginal delivery. Mine was for the bleeding that followed prostate skewering. How strange it all seemed! My partner was allowed in for a moment, and we exchanged looks of love and relief together with a brief hug. Fortunately, I had seen enough spinals to not be worried about the return of lower body function. Yet the experience gives a person immense appreciation for what it must feel like to be permanently paralyzed.

Once my blood pressure had stabilized, I was moved to the step-down unit, a more comfortable less intensely supervised cubicle, in which I was to remain until I could stand and void. My partner joined me, and we chatted some as I drank juice in prepa-ration for what I still hoped would be a quick exit. Three hours later, I was still there. I had been told that the catheter would be removed once I had sufficient sensation to find it irritating. I can only imagine what it must be like for those who have surgery and are catheterized for three weeks post-op. Return of function was definitely a slow motion experience. First the toes, right before left, a minimal wiggle, then some sluggish movement. Feeling gradually ascended like a curtain rising to reveal an old thawed self. My mind wanted the catheter out even before I felt it, and I began asking for its removal. It must be a challenge for a nurse to take care of a doctor when he's a patient. I was still pretty numb in my upper thighs and buttocks when I convinced the nurse assigned to me that I was feeling the catheter. She took it out and, based on my report, started to help me stand when she realized I was nowhere near as far along as I had claimed. Sheepishly, I continued to recline. After some additional time had passed, I was able to void and stand, but my partner and I knew I was still unsteady as I made my way from the waiting room to a taxi and rode the few blocks back to our hotel.

I had been provided with the necessities of recovery-pads, pain medication, coffee-type filters to collect any radioactive seeds that might get into my bladder and escape in my urine, a hollow lead capsule to dispose of such seeds safely, ice packs, and appoint-ments for an X-ray and a CT scan the following day. The very idea of a following day was something I could not process at the moment. I left the hospital a relatively happy man. Back in my hotel room, watching CNN headline news, an icepack between my thighs, I thought about dinner.

Chapter Nine

A Punch Absorbed

I was settled back in my hotel room. The next four days had been planned in advance. There is something very comforting about a plan. It suggests control and a way of encompassing damage. Having tests and a return visit to my implant doctor scheduled a day after the procedure made me feel things wouldn't be too bad. I should apparently be able to handle a whole morning of walking, sitting, and lying down on X-ray tables. There were further signs of hope. My appointments were to be on a Friday, the last day of the week, suggesting virtual certainty that I would feel up to them. The brachytherapy operation closes shop for the weekend. Would they schedule seed implants on a Thursday if there were a good chance some of their patients couldn't make it out on Friday?

I ate heartily and iced my crotch with frozen peas and ice packs, obligingly recycled by the hotel staff from their kitchen freezer. When I had to urinate, I stood at the toilet armed with my cone filter, tweezers, and hollow lead capsule. I remembered I was to trap and properly discard any stray radioactive pellets that might find their way into my urine. In the earlier high, I hadn't given the matter a moment's thought. Now I wondered, the first pee, how would it go? I had been warned that the stream might be quite wayward the first few times, and I was mentally prepared for pain as well. But the idea that I was now a vehicle for radioactive waste was something else.

A hundred seeds had been placed in my prostate in the most sophisticated game of darts imaginable. But darts they were, independent of the hand that launched them once they became embedded in their target. The prostate gland is not a uniform, homogeneous body but rather loose tissue filled with various exit channels. Seeds could migrate into veins and travel upstream to lodge in the lungs. They could escape through other channels into the urine. How would I react to finding a wayward pellet that I had to place in the lead container provided for disposal?

It took a bit for the urge to urinate to translate into the first flow, red from bleeding, and all over the place. I was happy that I was able to go and that there were no radioactive surprises in the filter cone. I returned the lead capsule to the top of the toilet. I was about to rearrange the pad that covered the puncture wounds when another little spurt caught me by surprise. This one wet my pants. I knew this would happen some time, but so soon? My mind struggled to accept this little mishap as a normal consequence of what had been done to me. However, certain occurrences are simply humiliating, and wetting one's pants is definitely one of them. It conjures forth images of incontinence, of old age, of babies in diapers, of little boys dancing at the playground trying to hold it in, or of severe and irreversible human plumbing problems. I knew better than to be ashamed, yet part of me was. I had screwed up in my impatience to get out of the bathroom. It was my fault, of course, because I didn't completely drop my pants and remain patient to the end. It could have been prevented, had I just been more careful. I changed my clothes, positioned the pad, cast the wet pants into the laundry bag as quickly as I could, and got back in bed, the ice pack on my crotch.

It was evening, time to take my medicine. Medicine has a way of wedding a person to the clock. The normal spontaneity of meals, drinking, and sleeping is often corralled into rigid schedules by medication requirements. Some prescriptions must be taken at certain intervals, others with meals, others on an empty stomach, still others cannot be taken in association with certain foods. Some interact with each other and should not be taken together. Some induce sensitivity to the sun. Some stain the urine creating hues that suggest bleeding. All can have side effects that may emerge at any time or may be imagined to have emerged. Once a person becomes dependent on medication, he becomes a scheduled human being. The timing and nature of meals may no longer be random. What is the meaning of an hour before bedtime if a person is accustomed to turning in whenever he feels tired?

While I was discussing my case with consultants, I had asked those familiar with seeds what I should expect. One person, the radiation oncologist who administered my external beam radiation, had said the aftermath of implants likely wouldn't be too bad if I "did drugs." When I asked him what drugs he had in mind, he mentioned two kinds, antiinflammatories and drugs that promote urine flow. It sounded like a piece of cake at the time. I knew I had a tendency toward acidity with ibuprofen, but there were newer versions that would minimize this side effect. The medication that promotes urine flow, Flomax, seemed to have a very benign toxicity profile, perhaps some transient dizziness on sudden standing, but not much else, practically speaking. When I left the surgical recovery area I had both of these in hand along with a four-day course of an antibiotic to discourage possible infection from the urine catheter. I also had medication to reduce the pain of urination. This drug, Pyridium, stains urine, clothes, hands, or anything that comes in contact with it, orange-red.

In medicine, we often speak of drug compliance. Sometimes, medications are given with the knowledge that patients will not be able to stick to the prescribed schedule or will forget to take doses now and then. As the number of medications increases, so does the complexity of interactions and possible side effects. If one drug causes headache and another possible nausea, what should you do if you develop a bad headache that leads to nausea? Every physical nuance, every bodily sensation, now has a tendency to register, to raise the question, is it due to the drug? I had no idea what "doing drugs" would entail until they were handed to me. One quickly becomes a prisoner to medication, dependent, nervous, and troubled by having to relate to these foreign substances entering the body at specific times. Even though I had received medication in the past for my cancer treatment, this was somehow different. The Lupron had been by injection once a month. The Casodex bombed and was quickly out of the picture. The Proscar was like an innocuous vitamin. Since the possible benefits of Proscar were long term, dropping or forgetting a dose caused hardly a ripple. Also, while I was taking these, nothing else had been done to me, and I was not trying to reduce a procedure's aftereffects.

If you have ever read a drug package insert, you know that medications are associated with a variety of side effects, the key factor being how often any one of these is likely to occur. I have spent my whole professional life looking up side effects in the *Physician's Desk Reference* (PDR) and prescribing appropriately. Every day, I casually write dozens of prescriptions, specifying quantity, timing, and duration without much concern about their impact. Many times I have simply said that side effects of a given medicine were unlikely, knowing that some of the side effects if enumerated, although rare, could be devastating. As a doctor, you cannot tell a patient all the potential side effects and still hope for compliance. Informing your patients requires a sense of balance and interpretation. If you casually mention liver or kidney failure, your patient probably will not take the medication, even if the chances are one in many thousands.

I have faced similar dilemmas when being asked about diagnostic possibilities. If a child comes to my office with a headache that has lasted three days, I am not going to list brain tumor as one of the possibilities when I discuss the situation with the parent. It certainly is on the list, but down very low. To mention it is to frighten the parent needlessly. If asked directly, I cannot deny the possibility, but I generally say something like "let's not even think about that" rather than responding head on. One would think that "yes, it is possible but unlikely" would be as reassuring, but it is not. "Possible" is much stronger than evasion.

An hour before bedtime, I took the antiinflammatories, the Flomax, and the analgesic that stained my urine. I avoided seasoned food so the ibuprofen did not cause heartburn and stomach pain. I avoided eating much dairy, especially as it interfered with the antibiotic. I planned that bedtime. I took care to wave, shake, and tap after urinating so I wouldn't stain my underpants if my penis slipped off the protective pad. I positioned and repositioned that pad to be as comfortable as possible. The pad's thickness, its backing, its ability to adhere to underclothes, its visibility, all became important issues for me in the coming days. How amazing is the human mind! A few hours before, I had been concentrating on spinal anesthesia and catheters. Now, I was equally concerned about underpants.

I waited for the pain and antiinflammatory meds to take effect and sought to sleep. My soporific was CNN headline news, a holdover from vacations in places with poor reception and limited station possibilities and also a habit from home. I awoke several times, beginning what was to become another ritual. I had to turn on the bathroom light so I could find the cone and the capsule and arrange and position myself. I dropped my shorts to the floor so they would be out of the way. I waited while my body registered its need and the urine trickled down to its exit. There was some discomfort and burning, but it was not awful. Eventually, a stream was produced, coming out in fits and starts and dribbles, taking unknown and unpredictable directions, sometimes splitting into two or more tributaries. The end was always uncertain. There was more or less a sensation that my bladder had not completely emptied. Nevertheless, things were working and the first night passed, frozen peas and ice repositioned until they became warm and the morning broke. As I watched my urine in the light of the early dawn, I was sure I saw bubbles, that is, air in the stream. What was this all about? What was going wrong now?

I don't remember getting up and getting dressed that day, though I made it to my scheduled appointments. Nor do I remember having breakfast. I already knew that caffeine was a bladder irritant, but I don't recall whether I took a chance on hot chocolate or settled for herb tea. I put on comfortable clothes and was off to my first appointment by 9:00 A.M. It felt good to be able to walk to the hospital that short block away, but I had to take my time getting there.

So there I was, back in the waiting room. And I waited and waited. After a while, it seemed I would miss both the CT scan registration and appointment time. My seed mates of the previous day were there also, one sporting a T-shirt stating the date and place of his seeding, a nice touch, I thought. Finally, I was ushered in to have a chest and pelvis X ray, and then I waited some more. The chest film was taken to see whether any of the seeds had broken away and traveled to my lungs. I had asked the "What if?" question, and was told the seeds were so small they hardly ever caused problems. OK, then why the X ray if there were no symptoms? I stopped second-guessing, reverted to patient status, and asked them to call radiology to say I would be late.

I waited a bit longer and was finally reunited with my implant doctor. He told me, with some satisfaction, that things had gone extremely well. Then he held up one of the X rays showing what resembled a little fireworks display within my prostate, and he proudly pointed out a seed lodged in a seminal vesicle. That was dandy aim or plain good luck, a beaut. I did not notice then, nor did I ever find out, whether that seed was placed on the right or left side. It would have been a stroke of special good fortune if it had been the right side where I had the most disease. On the other hand, the involvement of the seminal vesicles does not follow predicted likelihood very well.

I was told not to have sexual intercourse for several weeks. What a joke. Sex was hardly an issue, or even an interest at that point. I definitely didn't want to even get near my penis unless abolutely necessary. Moreover, my partner, having had a hysterectomy with removal of her ovaries didn't want to get near that thing either. In addition to all the tension and worry, first about her condition and then about mine, she was experiencing the consequences of estrogen deprivation. Her vagina was dry and intercourse was painful for her. The pleasure of sex is one of those imponderables. I think for many guys, the anticipation almost beats the act. The sex drive is strong, of course, when testosterone abounds. The desire is overwhelming as peak is reached, and your entire body thinks and feels that if you don't do it in the next thirty seconds, you're going to explode. You experience what Mother Nature tells you feels better than anything else in the world, and you experience it for minutes, perhaps a bit longer if you're lucky enough to be able to sustain the pleasure without exploding. Then you do explode. Then it's over.

I think it becomes a conscious effort for most men to experience much in the way of afterglow. The effort to capture that pleasure more often than not comes down to how many times could you do it over what period of time. But each time, boom and it's gone. It is only when that hormone is taken from you and you become a chemical eunuch that you step back and ask your-self, "What is all this fuss about?" Of course, you continue to go to great lengths to recapture it. And as soon as the testosterone returns there you are again, having at least the desire if not the ability.

My doctor and I subsequently talked about whether I would be sufficiently radioactive to place my patients at risk. The fall-off of radioactivity is so rapid that the risk may be judged mini-mal unless a child was to sit in my lap. Nevertheless, I expressed interest in lead-shielded underpants, which were available at a substantial cost. I would return later to try them on for size. I asked about the bubbles in my urinary stream. That was a con-sequence of the cystoscopy performed at the end of the procedure. The urologist had injected some air when he viewed the inside of my bladder. Yes, he should have forewarned me about the air, but I was a doctor after all. It often escapes doctors that many of us have become sufficiently specialized that we tend to have for-gotten medical knowledge that seems so common and ordinary to another specialist. I encountered this phenomenon frequently during my stint as a pediatric cancer specialist. None of us experts retained the facility and familiarity to diagnose or exclude an ear infection, the most common pediatric problem, simply because we spent our time looking at bone marrows, not eardrums. Of course, we all believed ourselves perfectly competent at this task, because as pediatricians, it was expected of us despite our subspecialty emphasis. It is better to deceive oneself and imagine skills we have lost, than it is to admit that we are only partial experts, not equal-ly competent to engage in all facets of our general field. Considering all doctors who care for children, pediatricians are more widely, but not more deeply, informed in general medicine than are pediatric specialists, while family practitioners are more so than are pediatricians. Generalists without specialties may know a little about a lot, perhaps tending to miss what is unusual. They may be apt to gloss over significant details more removed from day-to-day experiences. Good medicine needs both specialists and generalists, along with a healthy portion of humble pie.

My next stop was a meeting with the head nurse of the practice. Doctors prefer to sail above the nitty-gritty, especially when the news is unpleasant or its transmission is time consuming. I think I was with this nurse for about an hour, discussing the expected course and my follow-up. I should expect a honeymoon period of a couple of weeks, after the initial inflammation died down in two to three days. Then I would experience variable side effects from the radiation, hopefully mild, typically lasting two to three weeks. Would I be able to travel to Sweden a month later, I asked? Probably, she answered, but no guarantees. My doctor, of course, had expressed greater optimism on that point. We reviewed my medications and prescriptions were dispensed. I was given a diet that eliminated foods likely to irritate the bladder and prostate. The nurse advised me to stick to the diet both before and during the time I had symptoms of inflammation related to radiation. I didn't study the diet carefully then, but I did notice at a quick glance that it eliminated many of my favorite foods.

By now, I was quite late for my CT scan. It was raining, as always in Seattle, but fortunately the hospital had constructed a series of connecting aerial passageways between buildings. My partner and I navigated these corridors and eventually arrived at X-ray. Sign in again, and wait again. Scheduling medical procedures becomes an ongoing negotiation. If you have to wait for one procedure, you are likely to be delayed for the next. I lobbied and pleaded my case at the scheduling desk. I would be an add-on at the end. This post-op check was to assess the accuracy of seed placement. The CT scan would lead to a careful assessment of the degree to which the prostate had been radiated evenly, an evaluation of what is termed dosimetry. I knew in advance that the results would not be available until after I left Seattle. The tech was very nice to me, but clearly a bit put out by the delay and ready to leave after my CT was completed. Technicians have a difficult job. The work can be repetitive, the brief encounters with patients pleasant or trying. Their skill is often not appreciated by the patient who is in no position to assess it. The technicians are under pressure to resolve scheduling problems, and fit in emergencies. Friendly service is the only expectation patients have of technicians, and it cannot always be satisfied.

There were just a few CT cuts, so this procedure took only a short time on the hard gurney-like table. Yet I was sufficiently stiff and sore to need some help getting off that table and additional assistance putting on my shoes. I was a bit embarrassed by this. The experience made me feel like an old man. Able-bodied people become accustomed to carrying out basic acts of self-sufficiency and they take these for granted. To suddenly be unable to put on my shoes came as a shock to me. For a split second, I couldn't imagine a reason for it. Nothing was done to my feet. Why should I have trouble bending down? Then, to be unexpectedly dependent on a perfect stranger, someone with whom I would only have momentary contact, a pretty woman no less, and me a day after the assault on my sexuality. Suddenly, it all seemed overwhelming. I felt very bad inside. But in true guy fashion, I brushed off my feelings with an internal laugh and quickly moved on.

After the CT scan and a quick stop at the snack bar, we returned to the urology offices so I could try on the lead-shielded shorts. I was given more cones, then ushered into the underpants fitting area. The shorts were cute and cleverly made with snaps that allowed the lead blocks to be removed so they could be laundered. These were boxer trunks, which I happen to abhor, but the minor discomfort I associated with this style was rendered intolerable by the weight and bulk of the lead shield. When I tried them on, I was sure I looked and walked like Frankenstein. I would rather retire, I thought, then wear these shorts and I vowed to be careful and keep my distance from my little pediatric charges during the few weeks that a theoretical risk was present. All business now completed, we returned to the hotel and I rested, envisioning a relatively benign short-term future. Treatment was over now, and the consequences were completely out of anyone's control. Definitely time to hope and pray or whatever you do when you feel helpless.

We were expecting company. While still at home planning our excursion to Seattle, we had jokingly suggested to friends that they join us after the procedure and spend Shabbat and the weekend with us in our hotel room. Shabbat is the Jewish Sabbath, a day of rest when observant Jews refrain from work and activities that change the physical world. Judaism is defined by a way of life more than by a set of beliefs. We live by a code of obligations we take upon ourselves. Most of these are required of Jews alone. God, the originator of these obligations, is viewed as the organizing principle of the cosmos, a power we Jews hold to be purposeful, even if the purpose is hidden from our understanding. Whether the laws incumbent on Jews are observed or not is something every Jew must decide for himself or herself. Every Jew organizes his or her actions in relation to these laws known as commandments, living in close or distant relationship to what in Hebrew are termed mitzvoth. In this way of life, we introduce an element of care and reverence into every act, no matter how mundane. Derived from the touchstone of the biblical commandments, the laws that govern our behavior have become extremely detailed and they separate our actions from those who are not bound by the same necessities. As a result, Jews are often seen as being significantly different from everyone else.

Since we were observing Shabbat, we anticipated a bit of a problem as it begins Friday at sundown, and therefore would happen a mere day after my procedure. Observant Jews do not spend or carry money on Shabbat. They do not turn electric appliances on and off. They do not drive. All of these practices alter the physical world and are therefore off limits. And of course, those of us who observe also keep kosher, that is, we follow strict dietary laws. Our friends were also Sabbath observant. So we had to plan ahead.

The solution was to order kosher meals to be delivered to the hotel before sundown, which we did through the courtesy and kindness of the city's one kosher restaurant. Arrangements were made from home by phone and confirmed and reconfirmed several times. Our friends had driven up and were staying in a hotel about a mile away. They arrived a couple of hours before sundown, and we all waited together for dinner to be delivered.

In America, where the uniformity of "being an American" is a virtue and being different is tolerated, but not celebrated, observant Jews really stand out. Thus there is always a little tension when observant Jews find themselves out of their communities in the mainstream trying to balance their obligations against a wish to blend in as "normal" members of society.

Just before Shabbat, thinking I might run low on supplies, we hastened down to the corner store so I could purchase sanitary pads. I explored a variety of options, evaluating absorbency, how they might fit into my shorts, generate heat, or chafe my thighs. I examined adult diapers and pads located in the hygiene section. All of this was quite foreign to me, and no one had recommended a type or brand. The subject was glossed over, not addressed in any detail, almost as though it were taboo. We chose a bunch of panty liner and adult diaper candidates, and I took them home to try them out. Now I felt safer and properly prepared for future outings. As I carried my cache back to the hotel, I was reminded of ads for tampons, where a smiling woman was engaged in a sport surrounded by unsuspecting fellow players. I knew I would do my best to keep my fellows equally unsuspecting. Despite my needs of the moment, I could not escape some negative associations. It is my sense that many men harbor secret or overt antipathy towards women's menstruation and the necessities associated with it. They may see it as disruptive, a bother. They may associate it with PMS, interference with sex, or precipitous trips to the bathroom. A pity that this should be so, even for some, since menstruation is a normal manifestation of a woman's fertility. Thrust into an arena I preferred to keep at a distance, I felt awkward and out of place as I inspected packages ornamented with flowers, housing a variety of pads in different sizes and shapes. I definitely needed to be there, but I felt it ought not to be so. Surely, my feelings must have been heightened by my having been instrumented in the genital area. This is simply not an anatomic region like any other. We cherish and protect this part of ourselves and invest part of our identity in its normal functions.

Awaiting our Friday night dinner, I understood that there is something special about friends and community. We support each other and share our joys and sorrows. To be in the presence of friends was a real gift. Along the way, I had even derived solace from a childhood friend who lived 2,500 miles away, a friend with whom I have maintained contact for fifty years. We only spoke a few times throughout my treatment period, conversations filled with disbelief, empathy, and perhaps worry. Curiously, I found email to be a better avenue for this comfort than live conversations. Although he was distant and not really as available as I would have wished, my oldest and best friend remained a presence in my mind, and the connection itself was important. I imagined he was thinking of me and that if I asked, he would come to see me. The acceptance and neutrality of a close friendship is unparalleled. No one is as safe as a good, loyal friend. Two other good friends were closer to home. There was an extended group of friends with whom I was perhaps not quite as intimate, who nevertheless helped me feel supported. Men may not share intimate concerns with each other as much as women, but the feeling of closeness remains. I have an "honorary sister," my first pediatric colleague, with whom I have shared so many joys and sorrows. One very close friend, together with her husband, even offered us their home by the sea for periodic respites when my discretionary funds were at an all-time low. Her eighty-five-year-old dad, a world-renowned psychiatrist, became friend, advisor, and role model, having survived numerous operations, some for life-threatening conditions. Our local Jewish community provided support in the guise of people who were ready to cook meals, run errands, come over to chat.

One's immediate family also adds great comfort for a cancer patient at a time of fear or crisis. Family relationships are enriched by virtue of time, sentiment, and shared experiences. I was fortunate to have three special family members in my life when I needed them, though two of them could not accompany me to Seattle for the seed implantation. My mother, eighty-nine years old at the time, was still living independently, but failing health, hearing, vision, and memory all kept her at home. Her age seemed to leave her somewhat removed from the full impact of my condition, but she was a solid support to me even at a distance, alert to my moods and needs, a loved one on the telephone. She remains a pillar of strength to this day, despite her infirmities. It is amazing what just having a Mother still alive in the world will do to bolster your spirits when you are physically or emotionally threatened. My only child, a daughter, then twenty years old, was abroad and committed to remaining there during my procedure and recovery. She too was a great source of strength with her love, attention, and optimism. She provided me with hope for a future. A person has to have children to fully understand the power of that continuity. No other bond equals that between parent and child. My daughter's need for and appreciation of me were catalysts for recovery. I wanted to get well, not only because I still had a lot of life to live, but also because her life and my role in it were dear to me. After my procedure and in the days that followed, I was on the phone to both my mother and daughter. Knowing people were thinking of me around the world was especially comforting.

But it was my partner, my mate who actually shared the events with me as they unfolded. She was my source of intimacy, the person to whom I could confide my deep secrets and worries, provided I was prepared to do so. She shared the highs and lows as they occurred. She took care of me, saw every expression on my face, heard every nuance of my voice. She dealt with my cycling optimism and pessimism and helped me pick up the pieces where I faltered.

My partner and I certainly could have made it by ourselves, but having the company of good friends was a bonus we could not have imagined. And sharing Shabbat with two of them was very special. Dinner arrived. We ate in our hotel room and settled into the calm of Shabbat. The calm was marred, however, every time I had to void, grimacing when I stood up and sat down. I worried about each event, examining the quality and quantity of urine stream, assessing discomfort, checking crotch, pads, shorts.

The second night after seeds was not too bad. Our plan called for an outing the next day if I was up to it. An art museum was located just two blocks from our hotel. It was a slow walk, made awkward by the pad situated between my legs against my crotch. And it was hot and sweaty in there. I had to try to plan my bathroom trips effectively, since each was an undertaking. However, when the time came I gladly made the effort, because sticking to a plan is yet another sign of recovery. As it was quite boring in the hotel, I was up for the outing. I made it through the museum and lasted a little over an hour, moving from bench to bench with slowly increasing urgency as I became fatigued. There was one bathroom experience. I emerged unscathed.

The following day began with a tour of the city. Having lived in Seattle for three years, I guided the group around town, making a wide arc that took in the sites and views, stopping for a walk amidst the greenery at Volunteer Park, trying to make sure we got a glimpse of spectacular Mount Rainier. We walked about 45 minutes in the marshes alongside the lake opposite the university and took in the scents and flowers of the arboretum. This little tour further reassured me of my smooth recovery.

So far, I had proven my recuperation to myself by eating, reading, walking, and being a tour guide. The soreness, cones, and orange urine were becoming transitory footnotes, soon to be left behind. The stained clothes were but an aberration. The chafed thighs were a mere temporary annoyance. The pads were but an irritant, a reminder of treatment that was already in the past. I took my first bath and subsequently my first shower. I was on a roll.

My partner and I went to an art gallery by ourselves in the afternoon. We bought an old folio containing biblical passages in six languages, irresistible to my partner, whose academic background is in linguistics. A tangible reminder, such as a work of art, can arouse feelings of whimsy, sadness, fear, or confidence depending on its associations and the observer's mood of the day. I never gave a moment's thought to the continuing impact of a visual souvenir of my cancer treatment in Seattle, how it might affect me after the events surrounding its acquisition receded into the past. It turns out to be quite comforting. Its presence reminds me of the joy I felt when being able to go to a gallery was itself an achievement. It reminds me that happiness is often derived from simple pleasures, and that we should take nothing for granted.

Feeling good from the day's outing, we rejoined our friends for an early dinner overlooking the locks. We dined, watched the boats navigate the canal, saw the drawbridge ascend and descend for pipsqueak vessels with tall masts, and once again pretended we were just on that short vacation. The day passed relatively uneventfully. I took my pills, had my first bowel movement since seeds, experiencing none of the enormous pain I had anticipated, packed my bags in preparation for the flight home the next day, and went to bed.

We treated ourselves to valet service to the embarkation point for the bus to the airport. Considering all the things that could have gone wrong and didn't, it was almost comical when the bus pulled in twenty minutes late and we almost missed our flight. But we pushed as best we could under the circumstances and made it to the plane. A few hours later, we returned to the warmth and safety of our house, anticipating the pleasure of sitting outside in the garden and sleeping in the comfort of our own bed. Everything seemed to be on the mend. I had no further bleeding and the soreness was subsiding. On the fourth day after seeds, I stopped the antibiotic as directed. I also went off the analgesic, so my urine no longer stained everything orange. I was down to two medications, the antiinflammatory and the urine flow stimulant. I didn't need to filter my urine anymore and no seeds had escaped. I no longer needed those bulky, uncomfortable pads. It seemed I would soon be returning to my practice and resuming a reasonably normal life.

Fortunately, my colleagues had decided that I should take three additional days off before returning to work. I began to realize that I was tired, though I had no inkling that the smooth sailing would soon come to an abrupt end. I received congratulations and encouragement from friends and remained on a post-op high, a triumphant return home.

Chapter Ten

On Fire

I spent the first days at home resting, going to visit my mother, talking to my daughter on the phone, watching ballgames, reading a bit, and spending time with my partner. I went through my mail and tried to prepare myself to return to work. The initial days back at work were to be scheduled lightly. I move rapidly between examining rooms in my office. I usually move rapidly in general. But we all assumed I would be moving slowly for a while. In any event, I had to gear up for my first weekend on call. The first day back at work was fine, marked by congratulations and a warm welcome. I did well that first day, seeing patients, feeling good, careful to pee in the pot, sensing recovery in the wind. Toward evening, the soreness seemed a bit worse, but who could be surprised? I had been up and around all day long. I simply attributed the pain to fatigue and exertion. After dinner, I settled into a long warm bath and felt substantially better when I emerged.

The next day, I was more sore on rising, but I still did not pay much attention to it. Side effects could wax and wane, I had been told. Surely, I was just experiencing a bit of the waxing. As they day progressed, however, the discomfort seemed to be increasing. The soreness of the skin of my crotch was overshadowed by a new sensation. The area next to my rectum, sort of between my rectum and penis, but deep within, was aching. This inner ache was dull, not sharp or cramping. It did not become so severe that I wanted to roll over and die, but it was also not coming and going like a mere cramp. This was an exaggerated version of the short-lived pain I had experienced after the prostate biopsy. This was prostate pain. I also felt spasms both within my pelvis and at the tip of my penis whenever I urinated. Peeing had become a bit more of an effort, slow to arouse from the initial urge. When it came, it was painful throughout and afterward. There was no respite other than sleep.

It seemed way too early for the end of the honeymoon period, so I didn't know what was going on. By the end of the second day, I was dragging. Neither the antiinflammatory nor Tylenol seemed to make a substantial difference. I made it home and sank into a bath. This time, I popped a Vicodin narcotic to reduce the discomfort. I was up peeing during the night and it still hurt. But I dutifully appeared at work the next day despite the pain.

One of my colleagues offered to help out during my weekend on call. It's a good thing, because I was going nowhere. So I became a phone advice doctor, with my colleague waiting in the wings in the event someone needed to be seen. I spent more time in the hot bath. The urine stream became quite narrow, always splitting into two or three weak tributaries as the rate of flow slowed and weakened. I was having difficulty emptying my bladder entirely and would feel the urge to go just a few minutes after having voided. During the night, I had to stand for a while before the urine actually appeared and exited my body. All of this disturbed my sleep quite a bit so I added sleepiness to the daytime discomfort I was experiencing. Suspecting inflammation and bladder spasms, I now paid strict attention to the diet I had been given. Once I eliminated all the irritants on the list as well as the foods I was already limiting that seem to promote prostate cancer, I was left with very little to eat. It didn't matter at the time, because I was not very hungry when in pain. As time wore on, this diet would become a pain in itself and a recurring issue for me during the months to come.

Sunday night, I whipped off an email to my implant doctor asking him what he thought might be going on. There was no point in calling him. To reduce the acidity caused by the antiinflammatories, I added a drug that blocks it, Prevacid. These medications, the antiinflammatory and the acid blocker, entangled me in one of those phenomena in American medical care that makes any good doctor scratch his head in disbelief. Most insurance companies have drug formularies. According to price and who knows what else, they choose which drugs they will or will not reimburse. The choices are not uniform, of course, so different insurance companies reimburse different drugs. Drugs not covered require justification from the prescribing physician before they can be dispensed, unless the patient is willing to shell out the mega-bucks. It turned out that Prevacid, which was expensive, was not covered on my plan. My doctor could state that ordinary acid blockers were ineffective for me, but the process of doing so is enormously time consuming and frustrating for the doctor. It typically involves long telephone holds, forms, written justification, and the like. To avoid imposing on my own doctor, I bummed some Prevacid off my pediatric GI buddies at the Children's Hospital. Eventually, though, my doctor had to take care of it, and he also had to obtain authorization for Celebrex, an antiinflammatory less likely to result in acidity. That process took over a week and about half a dozen phone calls and fax requests. In this, as in all other medical matters, I had the advantage of being a physician and having a close working relationship with the people involved. My personal doctor was very accessible to me. The pharmacist was a man I had been dealing with on a daily basis for many years. These people were actively helping me, and it still took a week. When our great American health system bogs down and drags its heels in this fashion, it becomes an embarrassment to all of us. When the Almighty Dollar is involved, cancer and other health concerns quickly fly out the window.

After my difficult weekend, Monday dawned with a frightening experience. I was unable to void. I stood there, gazing longingly at the pot, waiting for the urine that never came. I tried relaxing. I tried to force it. Nothing. Finally, after nearly a half hour, I hopped into the tub filled with warm water, and was able to pee out enough urine to be restored to comfort. The episode upset me, as I recalled the experience of my colleague who had had to catheterize himself every night for eight months because he had urinary obstruction after seeding. It is a medical cliché that doctors have the worst complications of all patients. Was I to live out this cliché like my colleague? I am usually quite drowsy when awakened in the middle of the night. As my mind raced along hysterically, I tried to imagine having to catheterize myself at 3:00 A.M. The thought was almost paralyzing. Even if I were able to do it, how could I go to work? And if I couldn't do the procedure would I need an indwelling catheter for a few weeks? In that case, I certainly wouldn't be able to work and my vacation plans would be ruined. Having to cancel my trip would be a sure sign that I had lost control of my post-implant destiny.

After talking to my officemate, the one who had also had cancer, I called my urologist, and he scheduled an emergency visit that morning. He examined me, offered some reassuring words, had me drink some water, and did an on-the-spot ultrasound exam. Fortunately, I was not obstructed, just miserable. He attributed the problem to simple inflammation, perhaps some prostatitis, and possible infection. I should resume the antibiotics for another five days or so. The antibiotics could not be taken in conjunction with dairy products, not even with the milk in my coffee (which I was supposed to be avoiding). I also resumed taking Pyridium to reduce the pain of urination. This meant being back in those pads that kept the orange urine from staining my clothes, a small price to pay to avoid misery. I should increase the number of sitz baths. I could double the dose of Flomax. I was relieved. Just a little inflammation or infection, I thought, nothing to be concerned about. I went back to work and coped with the discomfort.

The story gets a bit awkward from here on. Partly, it is hard to describe sensations we may all experience differently. Also, because of societal taboos, I am tempted to skirt anatomic names for parts of the body, speak in euphemisms, and beat around the bush. I have obviously chosen not to do so. In reading about prostate cancer and its treatment, I found the single greatest deficit was the absence of graphic descriptions about how things felt. The pamphlets and information sheets handed out to prospective patients talk about pain, but do not describe it in detail. They will use terms such as "mild" or "moderate" and "operative site," but you won't read, "Your penis could feel as though . . . " Also, it is hard to recapture a specific physical feeling, even a painful one, once it is gone. I have seen this over and over again with pediatric patients, especially in those whom I treated for cancer. The children's anticipation of a painful procedure awoke generalized avoidance, some memory that what was about to happen was not a good thing. The procedure itself was accompanied by appropriate crying, thrashing, appeals to mommy or daddy, cursing with the older kids. But once it was over and the pain was gone, the smiles returned quickly, the children went back to previous activities as soon as they could and repossessed their typically cheerful and optimistic demeanor. Ask such a child to describe what had taken place and most would simply say, "It hurt a lot," then change the subject.

My crotch felt as though it was on fire. An ever-present dull internal ache seemed to sit like a stone on my rectum and near the bladder. My penis hung flaccid as though it objected to the onslaught and had gone on strike. Touching it anywhere was unpleasant. The tip of my penis was very sore, although no sores or redness were visible. This soreness, I later learned, can be referred pain from the prostate gland, but no one gave me that information at the time. "Referred" pain arises from one location, but is felt in another. Matters seemed to be getting worse daily. My doctor struck me as being somewhat surprised at first as he had assumed that my symptoms might be due to prostate infection that should subside in a few days. Imagine everyone's amazement when the urine analysis and culture, which should have revealed such an infection, came back normal! Now what was this all about?

My guy in Seattle urged patience. The voiding became constantly difficult and painful. Sometimes, I would stand there for ten to fifteen minutes and only be able to partially void the urine in my bladder, or not void at all, although I strongly felt I had to go. Other times, I would pace around, either in the bathroom itself or from the bathroom to my closet and back, over and over again, to achieve any result. It was becoming rapidly apparent that the honeymoon was over. This was radiation-induced inflammation arising at least a week or two earlier than anticipated. And it was severe, unlike the minimal discomfort described to me by my psychologist friend who had previously had the same treatment minus the hormones. Perhaps the course of hormones was making things worse? Or was it the palladium as opposed to radioactive iodine? As I contemplated the possibilities, knowing that none made any difference to my current situation, I also began counting the days to our departure for Stockholm, wondering whether I would be able to go. Fortunately, I still had three weeks to recuperate.

Along with my Seattle doctor, I sent an email to my radiation oncologist. He was a bit surprised, but mentioned that he had tripled the Proscar dose in a few patients with good response and no awful side effects. We also talked about steroids. These are medications that reduce inflammation. Most people think of steroids as the illicit drugs that athletes sometimes take. People with asthma are used to inhaling steroids as treatment. Anyone who has ever had an outbreak of poison oak or poison ivy may think of steroids as a lifesaver. These are powerful drugs with a variety of benefits and many side effects. Some side effects, such as heartburn or the development of ulcers, may overlap with the side effects of other medications. I was a bit leery of that, having some sensitivity in that direction. More importantly, steroids affect the immune response and can make people more susceptible to infection. I did not want to develop a urinary tract infection. I also got to the point where I just didn't want to add more medicines. It was all too much. There was much debate among my doctors about the steroids, one proponent, two detractors, one fence-sitter. The steroids might help a little or they might have no impact at all. I hemmed and hawed. Each day I weighed my symptoms. I was expecting this to last just a few days longer. I could handle it. I decided against the steroids.

This was evidently the "hump," the mysterious peak of radiation side effects, following which I should see gradual improvement. No one could guess how long my hump would last, whether it was to be a hump of days or weeks, or how much worse things might get. But clearly, in this regard, I was worse than average! What was I feeling? It is hard to recall specifically even though I definitely remember being miserable. During the daytime, I had to void frequently, and the urge to do so came suddenly and forcefully. Not only that, but a short time after voiding, I would feel I had to urinate again, and indeed, something always came out. When things were especially bad and I was back in pads to protect against stains, the orange still got to me. There was always a moment when I thought I had finished, but wasn't quite certain, and a drop or two would escape before I was resituated in the pad. We did a lot more laundry.

I was never completely comfortable. I had some rectal spasm sensations and occasionally felt that gnawing dull ache in my pelvis where I imagined the prostate to be. When I had a bowel movement, I often had to strain, and the straining aggravated my previous hernia site. The hernia had been repaired with a low-tension repair in which a mesh patch was sewn over the hernia bulge to contain it, but the defect that tore the tissue in the first place was not sewn together. I felt as though the abdominal pressure generated by my bowel movements might break the seal, causing the hernia to burst through, requiring further surgery. I did not want more surgery. It also just plain hurt. Fortunately, this urgency to move my bowels eventually subsided, albeit slowly and irregularly, and without the feared effect on my hernia.

Meanwhile, after my usual, busy pediatric day, and after being worn down by my discomfort and frequent bathroom trips, I had to face the night. I suffered weeks of sleeplessness. As they age, men commonly develop the need to urinate at night. We awake, feeling that our bladders are full, stagger into the bathroom, fumble for the lid, and pee. We then try to navigate between sleep and being awake during those few minutes, then stagger back to bed, hopefully avoiding a direct hit from that half-open door, and not waking the person lying next to us.

Now, because of the bladder and urethra spasms accompanied by the generalized inflammation, this process became much more complicated. When I awoke, my bladder not only felt full, it felt *full*. With the severe obstruction, urinating took a long time, but very little urine materialized. And I did not feel done. If I was truly exhausted and impatient, I would return to bed only to be up again, repeating the whole process about an hour and a half later. If I could manage to stay in the bathroom, I would produce more urine, but never enough to result in that sigh of relief that would indicate that I felt completely emptied.

This was the first week. As matters progressed from bad to worse, I found myself taking sitz baths and urinating while in the tub, because I was now standing even longer at the toilet without results. It's hard just to stand there in the middle of the night. I made the bath water as hot as possible, got in, waited, and eventually saw and felt warm orange fluid emerge from the tip of my penis. It typically took from fifteen to thirty minutes, after which I had to rinse off, get out, and dry myself before I could crawl back into bed. The combination of the hot water and the effects of the Flomax made me feel very light-headed. Sometimes I was able to go back to sleep. Toward 5:00 A.M., I often found myself awake and reading, resulting in a day that began with exhaustion.

It got a bit worse. I was no longer on antibiotics. My pills consisted of Proscar, the testosterone inhibitor; Flomax, the urine flow augmenter, at triple dose; Celebrex, the antiinflammatory; and occasionally Tylenol. The nights were uniformly bad. I developed a routine. Before retiring, I would sit in the tub and void. Then I would drain the water and refill the tub halfway with hot water only. The idea was that when I got up somewhere between 1:00 and 3:00 A.M., I would only need to add a small amount of cold water, if any to get in right away. Otherwise, it would take about ten minutes to get enough water into the tub to cover my pelvis when I was sitting there. Sometimes it was easier and more productive to sit. At other times, lying in the tub promoted greater relaxation and better results. Sometimes I wound up taking three baths during the night and a couple during the day. For a few days, I was so uncomfortable "down there" by the time I got home that I had to go straight to the tub. I don't know how I would have fared during a water shortage or if I lived in a place where warm tub water was scarce. Nothing else worked, and even if this provided only partial and temporary relief, it beat doing nothing at all. Except for the distraction provided by my daily routine, and by television and baseball games, I was entirely and completely focused on pee. The only time this was not true was when I was focused on poop—how loose, how hard, how many times a day, how much gas, how much pushing pain?

I always had the nagging pain deep inside my crotch and at the tip of my penis, but work's distractions made them tolerable. At times, I took a quick bath at home over lunchtime. Other days, I made it through to the end of the afternoon. When I was at home, I used ice packs. I sat on ice. I placed ice over my pelvis. Sometimes it helped, sometimes it didn't. I tried a heating pad too. Sometimes it helped, sometimes it didn't. Sometimes I slept with that thing between my legs. I went to see my pharmacist pal, and he suggested I try a rubber donut, that is an inflatable bagel-shaped seat cushion. I used it at home when I sat on a chair, but this did little to alleviate the penis pain and burning on urination. It did help when my tusch was sore.

Three weeks into this agony, my doctor assured me that I was probably at, or over, the hump and should begin to get better. Be patient, he again cautioned, as though there was an alternative. It was now about two weeks before our scheduled departure for

Stockholm. I began to doubt whether I would be able to make it. I limped along, recovering the best I could on weekends and on my day off work, which fortunately fell midweek. Finally, about a week before our departure date, things began to get better. The quantum leap occurred when I was able to skip the middle of the night sitz bath. I still had to stand for a while and add some judicious pacing now and then, but I didn't need the tub several times during the night. There were relapses, none predictable, none related to anything I had done or eaten, but on the whole, I was able to void. I immediately returned to having a glass of wine with dinner, and resumed my morning decaf. This was a milestone in my recovery. I hated that diet and craved the coffee!

As the inflammation died down, I settled onto another plateau. I was still unable to sleep through the night. But my risings were considerably shortened, so my level of functioning improved. Most nights, I was only up twice, or at most three times. I would hover over the toilet, lean my head against the wall and just stand there until it happened, trying all the while to remain sleepy. Then I would wait a few minutes and try to pee again, because I knew that my bladder had not completely emptied. Sometimes I was lucky and had a significant second void. Other times, I was not so fortunate and crawled back to bed knowing I would be up again. Many nights, this was just fifteen minutes later. I still had bladder spasm.

I had also begun having new trouble with bowel movements. They became frequent, not quite diarrhea, but accompanied by a lot of gas. Gas mixed with stool in the rectum creates distension of the bowel and makes you feel you need to go right now. The intensity of that feeling is hard to describe. Except for its being

one of your more unpleasant sensations, I would say it rivals the
urgency preceding ejaculation. The frequency and mushiness of
the ensuing bowel movements resulted in a lot of wiping, and this
led to a very sore butt indeed. Vaseline became a staple, as did
frequent inspection to make sure my underpants were not stained.
I think my walking took on a bit of a waddle, as it was quite
uncomfortable to move around. Sometimes I sat on the toilet
expecting enormous amounts of stool but produced only gas and
more gas, with or without little turds in between. I heard another patient describe rectal toxicity as being akin to trying to smile
with cracked lips, only it's the other end. That was very apt.

I sent another email to my doctor. In addition to the customary call for patience, he suggested Kaopectate and Lomotil.
So I added more medicines and was back to "doing drugs." Taking
the stuff made a difference, and brought this new problem under
reasonable control. But I still had my bad days, and they were
fairly unpredictable. A little too much broccoli or salad, and boom,
there it was again. My bowels seemed to have acquired a new
sensitivity to which I was not accustomed. Bananas and rice soon
became preferred foods.

As we prepared to depart on our trip, I collected a paper bag's
worth of medications. Although all these medicines might be
available in Sweden, the brand names would be different, and
obtaining them would be a royal pain. I took care to pack my
pills in my hand luggage so as not to lose them, but I had so many
that some of the more generic ones, like Tylenol, wound up in
my suitcase. I had already bought a plastic container, one typically used by the elderly who need to remember to take their medications. With four horizontal rows that matched the time of day

and seven vertical rows matching each day of the week, there resulted a grid of twenty-eight boxes. I filled a week's worth of boxes with everything I needed, and this little container became my shadow, not only for the trip, but for the weeks and months preceding and following the trip. It was not until I was down to just two medications that I could do without it. There were many days where I couldn't remember what I had already taken and when. It's the simple things that plague us.

The flight was uneventful. I managed to space my needs without difficulty. The Atlantic crossing was smooth, so my fear of being confined to my seat did not materialize. I even slept some of the trip. I had no diarrhea and no accidents, but I was very, very careful in the plane's lav. So there we were in Stockholm. I felt this trip was both a reward and a test. I think it is a good principle to have a pleasurable reward in mind when undergoing arduous and discouraging treatments. Short-term goals, even those that may seem trivial compared to the medical reality, serve to encourage us. We look to an end point, perhaps something we are ordinarily accustomed to taking for granted. A vacation or a birthday or finishing a project can subtly propel us toward recovery. There is always a hazard in raising expectations, as they may be dashed, but I feel the risk is worth it, and in my case, it paid off.

We stayed at a funky old hotel that was in the process of being remodeled. The construction struck me as a metaphor for the work in progress within my prostate gland. The side effects here were some noise and dust, but the hotel had charm, especially its ancient lift with its cast iron swinging door and heavy linked gate. I usually took the elevator, but occasionally walked the stairs. The beds were small, but adequate. The bathroom was one of those old European curiosities, but the plumbing was fine. However, the toilet, sink, and shower all occupied a single, small space, vented by a casement window that overlooked the court-yard. This set-up resulted in unforeseeable complications. The first was timing. My sittings often took several minutes. This deprived my partner of access to the sink, shower, and tooth or hair brushing. Conversely, if she was brushing her teeth and I suddenly had to go . . . And because of the uncertainties sur-rounding my bathroom activities, I was loath to use the general guest facilities outside our room. If we had to vent the bathroom, opening the window provided a panoramic view, both outward and inward. I had to close it to stand and pee in my special way. At night, the whole operation had to be conducted carefully by feel, since the door was hard to find in the dark. Of course, that was less of an issue than it first might seem, since it got dark around 11:00 P.M. and dawn broke about 3:00 A.M.

During the day, I did a fair amount of walking. Stockholm is an ideal city for exploration on foot. For greater distances, the public transportation system is superb and user friendly. A cen-trally located old town is utterly quaint and full of shops and restaurants, old buildings and narrow alleys. Museums abound, ranging from fine arts to old reconstructed ships. There are beau-tiful parks. Much can be seen by boats that take you to quaint islands in the archipelago. Stockholm proved to be an unexpect-ed tonic. I found myself able to do more than I had expected, which was exhilarating. This taught me that any reward we plan for ourself after concluding treatment should be attainable as well as enjoyable. Had I planned a hiking trip, I would doubtlessly have been disappointed. At one point, I even envisioned a side trip to Norway and long walks in the fjord country. My partner put the kibosh on this idea, suggesting that for a recuperating man, less might prove to be more. She was right.

I knew I was on the mend when I realized that with all the walking, my feet hurt more than my bottom. Imagine having aching feet bring you joy. I happily rested and soaked them, fully aware and appreciative of my good fortune. This was true recuperation. I was now certain that I was improving, and there was nothing left to do but await the return of normal functions and prepare for my first follow-up PSA. These two markers would settle my body's early response to all this treatment, balancing the initial result against the impact of the side effects. I could hardly wait!

Chapter Eleven

Steady State

I t took about four months to get back to normal. Of course, "normal" after seed implantation was not quite the same as normal before it. I still got up at least once a night to urinate. But most of the time, I had a reasonable stream, no pain, and could go back to sleep. The thin, multiple, spurting streams I had previously experienced slowly united, in short runs of success punctuated by periods of regression. My mind, now geared to recovery, noted the hills and valleys with corresponding elation or disappointment. After a while, the successes distinctly outweighed the failures. Each voiding session became less of an achievement test and receded to an appropriate place in my consciousness. Slowly, urinating reverted to a nonevent.

I still had sensitive bowels, and particular foods could give me diarrhea or that irritating combination of urgency, small, frequent bowel movements, gas, and occasional stains in my underwear. To this day, I carry an extra pair of shorts, just in case. I could now eat whatever I wanted, though it might mean taking a chance with my bowels, but the force of existing data made me a semi-vegetarian. Greens, squash, and pasta are all fine and health promoting. But what I really crave is a good steak. I love meat, but I now avoid it for the most part. Vegetarianism is probably less of an effort for those who are drawn to it voluntarily by conviction. When a diet is imposed or medically prescribed it can cause resentment. It is even more frustrating when you impose an unproven diet on yourself, one that may or may not be helpful to you, and one that runs counter to your preferences. What if someone showed that limiting meat made absolutely no difference to the outcome of prostate cancer or, on average, increased one's lifespan by six months? Would that be worth it?

I now indulged in soy in all its manifestations and guises—tofu, soy milk, soy chocolate milk, soy pills, soy burgers, soy sauce, soy pseudo-chicken burgers. If it looks like soy, it may be good for people with prostate cancer. Recent data also suggest benefit from a cup and a half of vegetables a day, especially greens, such as broccoli. On the bright side, green tea is a winner in this diet, chocolate is not far behind, and coffee is a distant third. There are a number of highly respected medical investigators conducting research on the effect of diet on prostate cancer prevention; these alterations in diet are not without some basis. However, increase the soy and veggies, increase the farts. If it gets out of hand, it's not only a personal affront but also a professional liability. I had to be socially acceptable, at least Monday through Friday. Many times I just snuck into the bathroom, gave thanks for the ceiling fan, and relieved myself of accumulated flatulence.

I thought myself a supremely rational physician. However, I added antioxidants, such as vitamin E and selenium; phytoestrogens, such as pumpkin seed oil; lycopene, a tomato extract; the green tea; and more recently, zinc. Some or all of these supplements may protect against prostate cancer. Why did I take them all? Was it fear and hocus-pocus? It is certainly strange to pop eight or nine pills at a time. Some are small, while others are humungous capsules that make you gag. I felt a little like a health food junkie. It was even more bizarre when I found myself talking to the staff at various vitamin and herb shops. Here I was, discussing the relative merits of one or another preparation with folks who had no medical training whatsoever, but expressed strong opinions about what does or does not work, doses, synergy, interactions, etcetera. What can they or anyone else know since there are no adequately controlled outcome studies, and most of the recommendations are extrapolated from animal or test tube experiments? Yet the preliminary data for effectiveness are enticing. Should they be ignored? Remember: With cancer, the clock is always ticking.

It was my assessment that one of two scenarios was fairly likely. My prostate might harbor residual, viable cancer cells. Or the process that led to cancer in the first place might still be operative and could transform healthy remaining prostate tissue into cancerous cells. I was drawn to the notion of making the environment hostile to these possibilities, thus retarding or perhaps preventing relapse. This approach, unsupported by hard fact, clearly comes at a cost—a monetary cost (supplements are not cheap) and a lifestyle cost. I decided that the changes were worthwhile, and I determined to live with the inconveniences they imposed.

Meanwhile, as the effects of the last Lupron injection finally wore off, some sexual interest returned. My partner had lost weight from anxiety. She was worried about it, but she looked great. I expressed my desire and we planned the event. As soon as I could, I had begun practicing in the shower, on doctor's orders, his sense being that after radiation, it was a use-it-or-lose-it proposition. It had not been enjoyable. It relieved no tension because there was no tension. It spilled no "seed" because there was none to spill. At that time, intercourse with my partner was not a reality due to her own medical problems.

I was nervous. It's that idea of performance. She reassured me that she didn't give a damn. I would be as dear to her as before, whether this worked out or not. We availed ourselves of all the extras that can simulate natural juices and get matters going in the right direction. There was much forethought, though not much foreplay. We did what was necessary to achieve erection.

With the first penetration came excruciating pain, not for her, but for me. The tip of my penis felt as though it was in a vice. The rest didn't feel much better. I had to withdraw immediately. There wasn't the slightest possibility of continuing. This was disappointing indeed. Remember, the hormones were coming back. I still do not know what caused the pain. My urologist shed no light on it. It felt just like the pain I had experienced after radiation, only more acute. Once I was out and lying on my back, the pain subsided immediately. I did not have this pain when practicing. Why now, I wondered? And why me? A couple of weeks went by before we tried again. It was slightly better, but it still hurt. I lasted a couple of minutes as opposed to a number of seconds. No fun here.

When we finally achieved success, it felt like a graduation party. I had made it. I could flip my tassel. It still hurt. It didn't feel that wonderful. It certainly didn't feel anything like before. The ejaculate was basically dry, just a drop or two. But there it was, leaving me with hope for the future. My partner couldn't believe I was so excited over this. As the hormone blockade lifted over these four months, things slowly reversed themselves revealing a kind of anatomic and physiologic spring. The pubic hair started to return and curl. My beard toughened—this a less fortunate consequence. The lipoma under my armpit softened and seemed smaller. Some of the guy sensations reawakened. I was attracted to women, although not as easily aroused. While things were still tenuous, I spoke with one of my doctors, the prostate specialist at my own hospital. He warned me that since the effects of radiation continue long after the actual treatment has ended, I might expect more erectile dysfunction in the future. I didn't want to believe him.

It was an appropriate time to try the V drug. This medication and others like it have become the source of much good humor. The jokes are great for those who do not depend on Viagra. Its reputation conjures up images of super potency, orgy-like wild nights, and never-ending sexual pleasure. Such notions feed men's fantasies. On the other hand, both in jest and in reality, there were reported consequences of excesses induced by the medication's effects, such as heart attacks and erections that would not go away. I took my medicine and waited. The peak effect is supposed to occur about one hour after swallowing the pill. What can I say? I felt weird, nothing I could hang my clinical hat on, just weird and spacey. My vision seemed a bit blurred and blues looked funny. My chest felt a little tight, but that may have been due to anxiety. The wonder drug seemed to work all right, but the erection was not sustained very long and I came quickly, the muscular pulsations almost resembling aimless twitches because they released no semen.

Sex has not been quite the same since then. I still enjoy it when it happens, or I think I do, and I certainly am happier with this than I would be with nothing. But a certain lighthearted joy and indulgence are gone. The wonderful thing about testosterone is that it promotes the sense that next time will be better, that all the old feelings and capacities will return, that eternal youth is not a myth.

Meanwhile, I had to direct my attention to more vital matters. I had been given a schedule that included a PSA six weeks following seed implantation. It would be my first one since beginning radiation three months before, and it would end the longest interval without a PSA since the beginning of my treatment. I was very tense, even a bit crazed according to my partner. I knew that the serial PSA determinations would continue to cause me tension. Each test resembles a game of never ending hopscotch. Emotionally, I was always teetering, trying to maintain balance and composure, seeking to see the next PSA as an opportunity for reassurance rather than as a death sentence. You are trying to get from here to there, hoping for a successful landing each time, knowing your reward will simply be that of remaining on one foot waiting for the next jump. You hope and pray, waiting for the test results, which may take a week or so if you are getting the ultrasensitive PSA. It amazes me that while I know the PSA simply reports what is going on in my body, actually what has been going on for months, I always see it as an instantaneous result and imagine my body jumping to the state of health reflected in that PSA. When the result comes in, I open the sealed envelope as if I were about to reveal the winner of tonight's Oscar. The anticipation is palpable, and the relief, if the result is good, overwhelming in its intensity.

For my first PSA, I chose the standard test, anticipating elevation due to my radiation treatments. I sweated those results, fearing they would be ambiguous. The PSA measured less than 0.1, its lower limit. I thought it better not to probe further by obtaining an ultrasensitive PSA to find out just how much less than 0.1. The next test would be due in six weeks. Time passes rapidly when you're playing PSA hopscotch. The second time, I decided to take the plunge and go for the ultrasensitive test. These were my decisions entirely. My responsibility was simply to obtain a PSA. This result was 0.04. I was starting to feel encouraged, in fact elated. When I told friends and relatives this result, I was almost boasting, as though it was my own achievement. Each good result called forth a little celebration—champagne, wine, an outing. I was reaching a point two fellow patients had related to me, a point I previously had been unable to understand. These men had each told me about their horrendous complications, one having had surgery and the other seeds, and then they had said they would choose the same treatment if they had to make the choice all over again. Suddenly, I was feeling the same way. The relief of having that low PSA, the feeling that treatment had been successful, erased the trauma of the side effects, especially since they had mostly subsided.

Six weeks later, another ultrasensitive PSA came back 0.07. Now ordinarily, such a result should be greeted with relief. After all, a "normal" PSA is said to be in the 1 to 4 range. However, after treatment, the range that is considered normal undergoes a shift. If you have had a radical prostatectomy, your PSA ought to be near or at zero. If you have had radiation, the comfort level is murkier. The decline is more gradual and the level that defines success is hotly debated. There are now anticipated bumps in the road, temporary elevations a year or two following treatment that do not mean relapse. This changes a previous criterion, which considered three successive rises in the PSA to mean treatment failure. It is unclear when to declare that a person has suffered biochemical failure, meaning a laboratory test that indicates relapse, well before a person experiences signs of disease recurrence. In many ways it's back to the very beginning, to that time when your urologist was first looking at your PSA trying to decide whether the value warranted a biopsy. The difference is that the numbers now being considered are much lower.

Why not simply do repeat biopsies or MRIs at specified intervals, you might ask? It seems that the distortion introduced by radiation and seeds makes tissues much more difficult to interpret than they were when the prostate gland was in its original state. Furthermore, since the process of destruction following radiation is ongoing, well past the time of treatment, it is hard to say whether cells that appear malignant are dying or still capable of growth and spread. Biopsies can miss areas of malignancy altogether, because six, nine, or twelve samples still represent a needle in a haystack if the amount of residual tumor is very low. And, even if we had a way of detecting microscopic areas of viable tumor, what should be done about it? Surgery following radiation is complicated and runs a very high risk of causing incontinence and loss of potency. Radiation following surgery is usually carried out if the margins are positive, that is if the surgeon couldn't "get it all out." Other forms of salvage treatment are as yet experimental, each fraught with problems or low success rates. When to intervene on the basis of a rising PSA still remains a judgment call. What is done at that point is often dictated by what is available.

Panicked, and with all this in mind, I wrote an email to my implant doctor asking whether I should be concerned about the slight rise in my PSA, and inquiring whether there was anything new, anything not yet reported in the way of hormonal manipulation, that might perturb any residual tumor cells in my prostate. Should I consider intermittent anti-androgen treatment? There had been some talk about continuing the Lupron injections for three years, but after my numbers were put into a predictive equation, it was determined that I fell into a category in which protracted hormone therapy did not seem beneficial. Should I consider it anyway?

I received the gentlest of reprimands from my doctor. Most of his patients, he said, would be happy to have a PSA like mine. I should neither worry nor obsess over small changes in the ultra-sensitive PSA. I should on no account impose the complications of additional hormonal therapy at this time. I was relatively mollified, and restricted my worry to low-level anticipation of the next PSA. On March 3, 2000, the result of that test came back as 0.00—none detectable! I was literally overjoyed and became tearful. There I was in my office, alone, with no one close by, having just received some great news. I quietly mouthed my thanks to God, once again acutely aware of the pull of the constant striving for life in the face of certain eventual death. I knew that I could not expect all future PSAs to remain at this level. How would I react to the next one, and the one after that? I was grateful to my doctors and to all those who stood by me. I was proud of myself for having stuck to my guns when making decisions. I felt I had made the best choice, although I will never know for sure . . .

Life has settled back to a kind of normalcy. Not a day passes by without my realizing that I have cancer. It is a chronic mental condition as well as a physical one. There are tangible reminders when some part of my body misbehaves. There are unwitting reminders in general conversation, in newspaper articles, on radio talk shows. Will I live to see a grandchild innocently pull this book from a shelf and ask me, "What's this?" Will I laugh and say something like, "Oh, that's something that happened a long time ago"? Prostate cancer, man's breast cancer, is rapidly becoming common, frustrating, frightening for those who must now anticipate its likelihood. A certain optimism has left me forever. I can no longer deny my mortality nor believe that I will escape the ravages of sickness and death by being a doctor. Yet the power of denial has not left me entirely. Although I know that I have this Damocles's sword hanging over my head, I do not live my life in despondency. I laugh at jokes. I watch movies and ballgames as before. I still manage to get upset over silly and inconsequential matters. I can still mount up a touch of road rage. In a given setting, I can still behave as though I were a young man, full of vigor and in possession of a seemingly endless future. There is, though, some sense of urgency over long-term goals and short-term desires. There is a feeling that time is being consumed at a faster rate than before.

I thought that my desire to receive compassion would lead to more compassion on my part, that my wish for more physician empathy would lead to greater empathy on my part as a doctor. I cannot say that this has happened in a dramatic way. If anything, I may have become a bit selfish and more driven to seek my own pleasure and fulfillment. Perhaps people who are basically satisfied with their life and work, as I am, will not undergo profound change after being diagnosed with cancer. Perhaps this life event has tempered my expectations. I certainly find that Good Health tops the wishes I give others and hope to receive myself. Aside from that, it is my sense that the changes taking place within me are subtle and yet continuously evolving. I am conservative by nature and by training, therefore not prone to dramatic shifts. I do feel, though, that my life and its purpose are being redefined, and I have yet to discover the nature and depth of the transformation.

I am aware that every decision I make carries this baggage. Professional and personal choices, my view of the future, my ideas about what matters in life, all have been affected by what has happened to me. I am more accepting of others. I am a little more self-indulgent. I want to enjoy things and not feel encumbered. I imagine places I want to see and things I want to accomplish before I die. I am sometimes depressed by the weight of what has occurred and experience a sense of fear and foreboding. Other times I feel that having more items on my agenda for the future will magically postpone my death. I may be troubled and envious when I see the young and romantic. I shy away from death in all its manifestations. My work and my family remain my refuge. I regularly retreat into the world of music, into my classical CDs, into the rhetoric and exuberance of the Baroque or the balance of the Enlightenment. I still wrestle with the concept of God, the idea of trust in a God, all the existential questions that have forever plagued me and that are ongoing grist for my mental meanderings. Seeing reports about supernovae, the human genome, various human disasters, all serve to put my life in proper perspective, but the effect is momentary. I return to a fully aware me, one that hovers between fear and awe, because I know that someday my life will end.

I continue to do what I can to stave off The Monster. I have continued to make my diet mostly meatless. I still eat more vegetables and soy. I exercise regularly. I try to find some enjoyment in every day. I take my vitamins and supplements. I hope for the best, and await my next PSA.

All is impermanent, the Buddhists tell us, in transition from one state to another. Our strong sense of "I" is just a mirage. Yet cancer is very personal and I cannot distance myself from it. I was not myself from the moment of diagnosis to the present and have had to painstakingly crawl back toward a remembered normalcy. I may never be quite the person I was before all of this began. Every day potentially provides a new emotional challenge, something I may need to integrate into my new reality.

If you are fortunate enough to have an intimate companion, you would be wise to share your various sentiments with that person. Tell your partner what you need, be it a kind word, a hug, a massage, a night out, a gift, or solitude. If you don't know what you need, say so. If you feel angry, say so. If you are frightened, say so. It is counterproductive to act out your feelings at the expense of your partner. You can pay professionals for that. Avail yourself of a therapist's services before you trample your supporters. Feel free to parry those who offer well-intentioned advice, those who exhort you to have a more positive attitude. Feel free to turn aside assistance that does not help you, but do not spurn the giver. Remember those close to you will also be experiencing fear and frustration. It is you who now need help, but this demands that you also be willing to be receptive and yield where previously you were dominant. Above all, let others know what makes you feel good and what makes you feel bad. They will not be able to guess your needs. Guard your close relationships, because they are bound to be challenged and threatened by this encounter.

Underlying the many negative emotions that I experienced was a current of will, determination, and optimism. A sense of hope offset my despondency. Prostate cancer can put you in a state of perpetual emotional bondage. You want to respect what you have and deal with it, but not be ruled by it. Fortunately, in the course of everything that has happened to me, I have been able to rediscover the hope, faith, and trust that things will turn out all right.

Almost a year after treatment, I close this tale with a final thought: Don't lose hope. Work to keep the monster in his box. Keep in mind the difference between "I have cancer" and "I am cancer." A well-respected urologist, a specialist in prostate cancer who also has cancer, has recently written that it is possible to be healed without necessarily being cured. Seek and find that part of you, deep within, that looks forward, that does mental and physical battle with anything that threatens to destroy you, that preserves your humanity, that nurtures your ability to live, love, and feel well. To every reader, especially to those about to embark on a similar journey, I say, GOOD LUCK!

About the Author

F. Ralph Berberich, M.D., has practiced general pediatrics in Berkeley, California for twenty years. He is on staff at the Children's Hospital Oakland and the Alta Bates Medical Center, where he has served as Chair of the Department of Pediatrics. Before entering private practice, Dr. Berberich was on the clinical faculty in the division of Pediatric Hematology/Oncology at the Stanford Children's Hospital, where he also served as the Director of the Hemophilia Program. He is a co-author of *The Available Pediatrician,* a guide to common childhood illnesses.